ABOUT THE AUTHORS

FORREST GRIFFIN is one of the top-ranked light-heavyweight mixed martial artists in the world. He won the first season of the Ultimate Fighter in 2005 and has been one of the most beloved UFC fighters ever since. He's a political science graduate from the University of Georgia and a former police officer, who can grow an awfully full set of muttonchops. But calm down, ladies—Forrest and his main squeeze, Jamie, live in Las Vegas.

ERICH KRAUSS is a professional Muay Thai fighter and the author of more than twenty-five books, including Anderson Silva's *The Mixed Martial Arts Instruction Manual: Striking*. He has written for the *New York Times* and is the founder and publisher of Victory Belt Publishing. He lives in Las Vegas.

D1167073

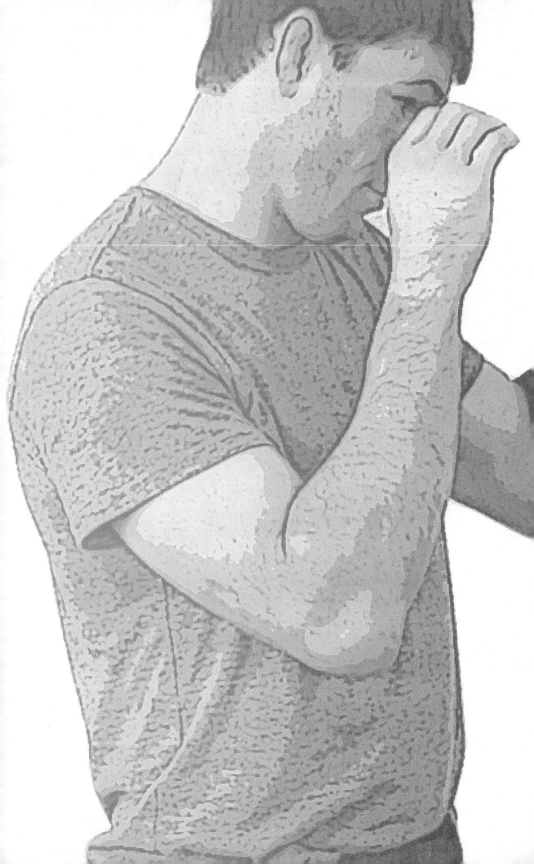

GOT FIGHT?

The 50 Zen Principles of Hand-to-Face Combat

Forrest Griffin

with Erich Krauss

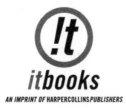

itbooks

AN IMPRINT OF HARPERCOLLINS PUBLISHERS

FIRST IT BOOKS EDITION PUBLISHED 2010.

Designed by Richard Oriolo

Library of Congress Cataloging-in-Publication Data has been applied for.

ISBN 978-0-06-172172-4 (pbk.)

10 11 12 13 14   WBC/RRD 10 9 8 7 6 5 4 3 2 1

To my stepfather, Clifford Abramson, for teaching me how
    to be a man.
To my beautiful wife, Jaime, for putting up with me.
To Mike Pyle for being the best cornerman in the world,
    which is much like being the best bridesmaid in the
    world.
To Byron Danielson for being able to figure anything out.
To the letter *q* (lowercase only) for being exotic.
To John Wood for defining the stereotypical Vegas
    douche bag, yet still being a great guy.
To Mark Beacher for having cool tattoos.
To Randy Couture for being an inspiration to old folks
    everywhere.
To James Roday for being clever the way I want to be.
To Bob Saget—enough said.
To Mike Whitehead for being a tank.
To broccoli for smelling like farts before you eat it and
    being difficult to spell.
To Hollywood for somehow making it cool to be Irish. It's
    getting so popular, in fact, that we're thinking about
    making a move on the Jews.

Special thanks to Paul Thatcher for the photographs
that appear in the insert.

Special thanks to Bret Aita for
his editing genius.

Special thanks to everyone at Zinkin Entertainment
for all of their hard work.

Special thanks to Eric Hendrikx
for shooting the technique photographs.

Many of the names, places, and even facts in this book have been changed to protect Forrest Griffin from getting sued by a bunch of douche bags. Very few small animals were harmed during the making of this book. The ones that were harmed were not in the "cute" category, so it's all good.

A NOTE FROM THE PUBLISHER

We and Forrest had some harsh verbal *and* physical altercations in the course of selecting a title for this book, which is obviously *Got Fight?* (If you missed it, we wouldn't go admitting that to anyone because it's on the damn cover.) Forrest is a formidable opponent—one with devastating leg kicks, sick submissions, and a jaw like a cast-iron stove, but *we* bite and he tapped out, and we got our wish—to call this book *Got Fight?*, which we think is pretty friggin' provocative. But we did agree to note his objection in the beginning of the book. Here is a phone message Forrest left for his editor on New Year's Eve 2009 (we suspect that alcohol was involved):

> I hate to beat a dead horse but you sound like a woman on your fucking little answering machine there. This is Forrest Griffin, as you can tell I'm from fuckin' Georgia—not just Georgia, FUCKIN' Georgia. *Got Fight?* is not a good title for me. Look, the whole "Got Milk?" thing was 1994. I actually Googled that shit. Nineteen ninety fuckin' four. It's more than a decade past, brother, so, uh, we're going to come up with a new title and you're going to develop a manly voice like mine [dark, raspy laugh].

Publisher's rebuttal: "Got Milk?" is still alive and well and milk builds strong, healthy bones, just like Forrest's.

Here are *Forrest's* titles, big, tough creative guy that he is:

Who Moved My Nose? (his favorite)

Fist Meets Face

Death Is a Journey and My Bags Are Packed—The Forrest Griffin Story

Punch Drunk

Face Full of Scars

A Few Scars More (assuming we do a sequel)

CONTENTS

ACKNOWLEDGMENTS   xv

YOU *MUST* TAKE THIS TEST BEFORE READING *MY* BOOK   1

BOOK 1 **THE PHYSICAL**   13

BOOK 2 **THE MENTAL**   61

BOOK 3 **SMART ADVICE**   99

BOOK 4 **HANDLING YOUR BUSINESS**   127

BOOK 5 **42 FIGHTING TIPS**   135

BOOK 6 **THE VAULT OF SUPERSECRET TECHNIQUES**   171

EPILOGUE   189

ACKNOWLEDGMENTS

For some reason, writers like to thank people at the beginning of their books. I understand if the book is really good, like Hemingway good, but what if the book sucks? I'm pretty sure that the book you are currently holding will only make you stupider, and I don't want to insult anyone I care about by putting them in the acknowledgments. It would be like dropping a turd into a napkin, setting the greasy bundle on the shelf in a bookstore, and then calling home and saying, "Hey Mom, just wanted to thank you for making the dump in a napkin possible." I tried backing out on the acknowledgments altogether, but my publisher used a bunch of big words, like *foreclosure of guilt*. He said he didn't want people to know the book was a turd in a napkin until after they bought a copy. I then tried to thank a bunch of people I actually hated, you know, to insult them by being associated with this book, but I got shut down (thank you, Satan; thank you, "guy who beat me up in the fourth grade," and, thank you, hot chicks who laughed at me in high school). So, I guess I have to thank some of the people I really care about. If you happen to be one of those people (and I'm sure you are, because what kind of idiot actually reads the acknowledgments to a book), please, please forgive me.

First and foremost, I would like to thank my mother for pulling me out of the Georgia public school system. It would have been nice if she could have done it before I got my ass kicked forty thousand times, but I guess later is better than never. I would also like to thank Kevin Garnett's mother because she, too, seems to have done a good job. Next, I would like to thank Adam and Rory Singer of the Hardcore Gym. Rory is an awesome friend because he never lets us get overcharged for anything. If we go to eat and our bill is five cents too much, he'll raise hell. It doesn't matter if the waitress only weighs a hundred pounds, he'll fight the bitch right there on the spot. Adam is the world's best grappler in the state of Georgia for a period of two or three minutes. After those two or three minutes, he gets up and has a soda—*Oh, you've almost got that submission, Forrest, think it's time to grab a Coke . . . Oh, I'm sure you could do a lot from that dominant position, but you got to get off me because I'm having an asthma attack. Best go get a Diet Dr Pepper.* In addition to showing me the tricks of the grappling trade, he has also been my primary source for reading recommendations. He's the guy who turned me on to *Fight Club* before the movie came out. I also admire him for the direction finder built into his head. Under the influence of extreme amounts of alcohol, he not only has the un- canny ability to find the rent-a-car, but he can also take us from any strip club back to the hotel. Seriously, every one in the car could be completely lost, and he just points off into the darkness of night and goes, "I think home is some- where over there." Everything about the guy is impressive, but his biggest ac- complishment to date is inventing the acronym MILF. Some people might doubt this, but swear to God, he was using that shit ten years before *American Pie.* And to Raffi A. Nahabedian for putting this whole deal together, and for mak- ing me a big famous author.

The last guy I would like to thank is my editor, Adam Korn. Originally, there were twenty editors who wanted to work on this book, but he bested all of them in an illegal cage match. I just recently learned that 90 percent of edi- tors are women, so I'm not sure of the kind of competition he faced, but I can honestly say this book would not have been written without him. Adam Korn is a unique martial artist in that he's not fat, forty years old, and into brainwash- ing kids. He understands the mind-set of a fighter and helped shape, write, and edit this book from beginning to end. (Fuck you, Adam. I want the thirty-eight bucks you promised me for writing this horsecrap acknowledgment. I'm com- ing for you, bitch. I'm coming!)

YOU *MUST* TAKE THIS TEST BEFORE READING *MY* BOOK

All the really cool roller coasters of the world require you to be a certain height to experience their awesomeness. In no way is my book as cool as a roller coaster, but nevertheless, I have imposed a restriction on those of you who are attempting to read it. I don't give a shit about how tall you are or how much you weigh. I don't even care if you're into really weird shit, like burning your nipples and stuff. All I care about is your manliness. I mean, how would it make me look if a bunch of sissies were reading my book in between their pillow fights? Not too good, that's how. So before I fill that empty brain of yours with all sorts of smart things, I'm going to give you a test, much like the tests *Cosmo* gives to women. And shut the fuck up about how I know such tests exist. It's called research, dumb-ass. So anyway, instead of testing whether or not your lover is worthy, I'm going to test your testosterone levels. If you're a woman, I don't want to hear your sniveling. There are a lot of women out there who are manly, so you best sprout a hairy sac in a hurry. This book is about guy shit.

Now, if you score forty points or above on the test, feel free to walk tall, brother. You are indeed a real man, and I have no problem with you absorbing the knowledge on the coming pages. If you score between thirty and forty points, you've got some chest hair to grow. I'll still let you read my book, but it must be done in the privacy of your own home. If someone should ask you if you read my book, you must say, "No, I tried, but it is far too manly for me to comprehend." If you score below twenty points, put my book down immediately and back away from it slowly. As a matter of fact, you might as well slip into a pair of panties, slap on some lipstick, and learn how to become a really bad driver because there is no hope of you ever becoming a man. No one is watching you take this test, sister, so you won't be doing anyone any favors by cheating. Just so you know, chicks cheat on these kinds of tests all the time. When asked if their man's love stick is large enough, they always check "no." Lying bitches. The reason I bring this up is that a real man never follows in the footsteps of a woman, so if you cheat, you are not only unmanly, you are also going to hell. Seriously.

#1 You wake up one morning to find a really fat chick lying next to you in bed. How do you react?

    a) You somehow convince the Woolly Mammoth to squeeze out your bedroom window so no one sees her leave, remove the wiry hair from between your teeth, and never tell a living soul about what you have done.

    b) Have her leave through the front door, but make up a bunch of excuses about how you were too drunk to get it up when your buddies start busting your balls.

    c) Take her out for breakfast and nod "what's up?" to your friends when they give you funny looks. You don't go so far as to lick the syrup off her lips at the end of the meal, but you smile and treat her with respect.

    d) Thank her for taking your virginity and nervously ask her for her phone number.

    e) Do not wake her up. Just leave your home and never come back.

ANSWERS

    a) +0 points. Let me break this down for you. Sleeping with a fat chick is an automatic –5 points, but covering up the dark moments of your life like an old-school vet is definitely manly, earning you +5 points. If you should ever find yourself in this scenario and react in such a manner, consider it a wash on the manliness scale.

b) –10 points. In this scenario, you get –5 points for sleeping with a fat chick, and then you get another –5 points for being a whining bitch.

c) +5 points. If a real man slips in a pile of dog shit, rolls down a hill into a puddle of pig shit, claws his way out only to be shit on by a cow, he still climbs to his feet with pride. Sleeping with a fat chick and holding your head high is the same type of scenario. It requires balls of steel and an unbreakable sense of pride, earning you +10 hard-earned points of manliness. Subtract the five points for the deed itself, and you end up with +5.

d) +0 points. If this was your answer, the reason I didn't award negative points is that I am now going to ask you politely to stop taking this test. All real men lose their virginity to prostitutes. However, if the fat chick in question was indeed a nighttime model, I will let you slide with zero points and a warning.

e) –15 points. You are a coward, and cowards aren't manly.

#2 Which do you shave more, your face or your genitals?

a) Face.

b) Genitals.

c) Never shave either.

d) Shave both equally and at the same time.

    1) *Face and then balls.*

    2) *Balls and then face.*

ANSWERS

a) +0 points. Shaving your face makes you a man but not manly.

b) –5 points. You're disgusting. I should have taken away 10 points.

c) +10 points. You probably live in the hills and kill things, both of which are ultramanly. If you have some type of wild animal as a

pet, such as a badger or wombat, give yourself an extra +5
points. And if you actually have a girlfriend (has to be a woman,
not the badger or wombat), give yourself an additional +5.

d) +0 points. When you're in the shower with a razor, giving both
your face and sac a "once-over" is not manly or unmanly. However, the order in which you do the shaving is very, very important. If you shave your face and then your balls, as long as you
dispose of the razor afterward, give yourself +5 points. If you
shave your balls and then your face, it means that you secretly
like the scent of nut sac and you are not in any shape or form a
real man. As a matter of fact, go ahead and give yourself –15
points.

#3 How much does your favorite pair of jeans cost?

a) $200 or more.

b) Between $100 and $200.

c) Between $50 and $100.

d) Under 50 bucks.

ANSWERS

a) –15 points. Real men don't pay that much for a washing machine
or their hookers.

b) –10 points. $150 is a brand-new chain saw.

c) –5 points. Real men are frugal. They are cheap with their beer
and food, so what the fuck makes you think they'd spend that
kind of money on jeans?

d) +10 points. Give yourself an extra +5 points if that favorite pair
of jeans has an oil stain on them.

#4 Your friends take you out to an all-you-can-eat buffet for your thirteenth
birthday, and then surprise you afterward by taking you to Dollywood for
a little bungee jumping. You're just a kid, so you don't see how bungee
jumping after an all-you-can-eat buffet can go terribly wrong. You think

that perhaps you might throw up, but instead you shit yourself. Remember, you're just a kid. How do you handle the situation? Seriously, I want to know.

a)   Jump in the nearest public pool.

b)   Pretend nothing has happened and go about your day.

c)   Go to the public restroom, remove your shit-soaked boxers, and throw them in the trash can. Next, remove your socks, dampen them in the sink, and then clean up everything your boxers didn't catch. Once you're done, dispose of your socks. When you get home and your mother asks what happened to your socks, tell that nosy bitch to mind her own business. Afterward, go upstairs and cry yourself to sleep.

ANSWERS

a)   +5 points. Although real men don't drag others down when their ship sinks, they are quick problem solvers. If the pool is twenty feet from the location where you did the shitting, give yourself +5 points. However, if you walk all the way home and then jump into your neighbor's pool, give yourself −5 points . . . unless your neighbor is an asshole who never invites you over to go swimming.

b)   +5 points. As I previously mentioned, real men always keep their chin up. If they have shit in their back pocket, they have shit in their back pocket. Deal with it.

c)   +0 points. The reason I didn't give negative points for this reaction is that shitting yourself at Dollywood is a tragic experience that no child should have to go through on his thirteenth birthday. It's absolutely terrible. Your friends constantly make fun of you, and it's not until much later in life when you become a fighter or something of that nature that you finally begin to earn just a shred of respect back from them. I don't care if it's not manly—I give a pass to every thirteen-year-old who shit himself at Dollywood while bungee jumping and then had to live with the horrible repercussions for years to come.

#5 You go on a first date with a respectable, attractive woman. How do you handle it?

a)   You pay for everything, open doors, and kiss her good night instead of trying to get into her pants.

b)   You tell her that she can order the most expensive thing on the menu and that you're picking up the check.

   1)   The most expensive thing on the menu is a $60 steak.

   2)   The most expensive thing on the menu is a Big Mac.

c)   You focus on how broke you are during dinner conversation and talk her into paying the bill.

d)   The moment you pick her up, you ask for gas money.

ANSWERS

a)   **+10 points.** New-school manliness cannot contend with old-school manliness. If you're a gentleman like Clark Gable, you are a real man. However, if you try to fuck your date at the end of the night, you get zilch. With this one, it's all or nothing.

b)   **−5 points.** Unless you've got old-school manliness, never offer a woman the most expensive thing on the menu. By saying nothing, you can tell what type of woman she is. If she orders the most expensive thing on her own, she is most likely out for your money. If she orders the cheapest thing on the menu, she probably lacks confidence and will be easy to bed.

   1)   If you're at a really nice restaurant where the most expensive dish costs $60 or more, you're an even bigger douche bag. Go ahead and subtract another 15 points.

   2)   If you took your date to McDonald's and she actually walked into the place, you already know she has no self-respect. In such a case, offering her the most expensive thing will probably make her happy and horny. Consider it a wise move and give yourself +15 points.

#6 You just got knocked the fuck out. Joe Rogan comes over and asks you what happened. What do you say?

    a)   You immediately begin making excuses. Tell everyone how your hand was hurt going in, your wife left you, you got the flu. Just rattle off every bullshit reason for the knockout you can think of.

    b)   You don't say anything because you are too busy crying.

    c)   You say, "Everything was going good, and then I just got knocked the fuck out."

ANSWERS

    a)   −10 points. Real men don't make excuses, even when those excuses are legitimate.

    b)   −5 points. The reason I didn't subtract more . . . well, you know the reason.

    c)   +10 points. This is the way every loss should be handled. In addition to making more fans, you don't go home feeling like a jackass.

#7 In a raffle you recently won a gigantic douche-mobile, such as a Range Rover, Hummer, or some kind of lifted truck. What do you do with it?

    a)   Go off-roading without worrying about scratching the paint or acquiring a few dents.

    b)   Donate the piece of shit to charity.

    c)   Trick it out by purchasing fancy rims that turns it onto an on-road vehicle only.

    d)   Use it to haul tools and lumber back and forth to work.

ANSWERS

    a)   +5 points. In order for off-roading to be extremely manly, you have to do it in something that isn't built for the dirt, like a Honda Civic. But showing that you don't care about the appearance of the vehicle gives you +5 points.

    b)   +10 points. I mean, come on, who really needs a Hummer.

c)   −75 points. Do I really need to explain?

d)   +10 points. Real men have manly jobs, and sometimes those manly jobs require a big vehicle. Gardening tools don't count. You've got to carry big tools, like lathes and grinders and wood splitters. . . . And no, I don't really know what a lathe is either.

If you passed the test with the appropriate number of points, feel free to consume the coming wisdom. If you did not pass the test, I feel sorry for you. However, being the nice guy that I am, I will attempt to improve upon your manliness by giving you some tips. Once you've committed these tips to memory, you must put the book down and go practice. After two years and nine days have passed, you are free to pick the book back up and take the test once again. Good luck (jackass)!

One More Thing Before We Get Started: You *Must* Improve Your Manliness

Most people have the completely wrong idea about what it takes to be a real man. If your goal is to attain a heightened state of manliness, and someone has been feeding you the wrong information (i.e., your chick or mother), you need to follow the guidelines set forth below. Personally, I'm a man's man. I say this because on many occasions I've been explicitly told that in no way, shape, or form am I a *ladies'* man.

The Real-Man Checklist

Repairman: A manly man knows how to fix shit. If the heater is on the fritz, he knows how to take it apart and put it back together. The more cusswords you use while doing the repair job, the more manly you become. It also helps to show at least three inches of butt crack and fart regularly.

Mechanic: Most manly men know how to fix cars, but it is not mandatory. However, you need to have a basic understanding of what's going on underneath the hood. If you have a friend who claims to be a man, yet he can't tell you what an alternator does or identify it, he is not a man.

Beer: All real men drink a specific brand of cheap beer. While I was growing up, my stepfather, who was the manliness man on the planet, drank Schlitz tall boys. There was no room in the fridge, so he just left them on the counter and drank them warm. One day I asked him why he drank Schlitz, and he said, "It's only 3.1 cents per ounce. Beer is an acquired taste, so you might as well acquire a taste for cheap beer." That's some manly shit.

Chef: A lot of people feel real men should leave the cooking to women, but that is complete bullsquash. Real men cook all the time, but there are some strict guidelines. First, all cooking must be done on a grill, even during winter. *Especially* during winter. Second, you can't cook anything fancy. Stick to meat. Third, you can't use too many condiments or know the names of the seasoning you used. If someone asks you what spices you put on the chicken, you must reply, "Hell, I don't know. It came in a package."

Intelligence: Real men don't need to be particularly intelligent about general matters, but they do have to be smart when it comes to guy shit. First and foremost, they must know the military ranks in order—corporal, sergeant, lieutenant, etc. If someone says something about a full bird, and you think it's when you elongate your middle finger, which is what I thought as a kid, then you're not a real man. I would suggest writing down the military ranks so you can study them, but real men don't write. (Note: I'm a man because I broke my own badass rule to write this book, which tells all *you* assholes to not even *start* writing. . . . Does that even make sense?)

Hunter: In order to be a real man, you don't need to be a lumberjack who lives in the woods. You also don't need to kill your food with your own two hands (though it certainly helps). At least once in every *real* man's life, he has killed something, cleaned it, and then consumed it later that same day. Shooting a buffalo and then losing track of it in the forest or paying someone to stuff it doesn't count. You must kill, clean, and eat. There is nothing quite like the steamy, meaty smell that emanates from a freshly dressed carcass.

Ways to Lower Your Manliness

Hair Removal: If you shave your chest, or God forbid any other part of your body, more than you shave your face, you are not manly. You're hygienic, but not manly. Although I have to admit (and I would have never pictured myself ever saying these words) I actually *prefer* to roll with guys who shave because I end up with less of their body hair in my mouth. But note, I tend to look down on them. You're also not a real man if you get electrolysis; I don't care how many tattoos you get—you'll never be manly. Now, if you shave your chest to get women and feel you deserve a partial pass, you're wrong. Why in the world would you do that? A real man never caters to women.

Tanning-Bed Membership: If you pay monthly dues for a tanning-bed membership, you bear no resemblance to a real man. I say this because when guys tan they usually put their junk in a sock or cover their package with a washcloth. This is disturbing, not manly.

Self-Help Books: The act of reading one of these types of books (unless Forrest Griffin happens to be the author—because *he* has *perspective*) is, in and of itself, a womanly deed. Briefly scanning, spot reading, or faking the reading of these books is, however, an acceptable method of conflict avoidance when dealing with a relentless, pesky wife or girlfriend; but actually completing these books means that you are either such a bitch of a man that you are succumbing to the will of your female master or your testosterone is leaking out your nipples. In any case, consider yourself warned.

Examples of Real Men

Bret Favre is my favorite real man right now. He's got a fucking Levi's commercial, and that's some manly shit right there.

Ernest Hemingway was a real man, and then he killed himself, elevating his manliness to new heights. You hear what I'm saying, pig licker?

David Caruso from *CSI Miami* is a real man, and I'll tell you why. This guy has absolutely nothing going for him. He's a skinny, ugly, redheaded dude who looks like he would break in half if you hit him, yet he walks with a swagger that convinces you he isn't afraid of anyone or any*thing*. That swagger makes him a real man.

Clint Eastwood is obviously the epitome of a real man. If you feel you're a real man and try to compare your manliness to his, you're stupid.

The old Chuck Norris used to be a real man. I'm not quite sure what happened to his manliness—perhaps it has something to do with two hip replacements and the fact that he dyes his hair.

THE PHYSICAL

The Devil Wears a
Pocket Protector

The toughest dude on the planet is not competing in the UFC or any other MMA organization. He doesn't train in the martial arts, shoot roids into his ass cheeks, or even hit the heavy bag. He couldn't have. From the looks of him, it's impossible. I don't know his name or what he's been up to for the past six years, but I'll never forget his face.

Back when I was attempting to play football for the University of Georgia, I'd occasionally catch a ride with a group of meatheads who were also attempting to play football. One afternoon, four of us were packed into a Jeep with the top down, cruising around for a while, when someone had the bright idea to go down to Georgia Tech and harass some of the smart folk. With nearly a thousand pounds of muscle, fat, and attitude weighing down our ride, we trolled around campus. I wasn't exactly sure what my cohorts had in mind until one of the guys jumped out of the Jeep while it was still rolling and headed straight for the only person in sight. The target happened to be the biggest geek I had ever seen. Now, I'm not calling this kid a geek because he had more brains than all of us combined and actually *went* to class, but he was five nine, packed at best a hundred twenty pounds, wore a button-down shirt, and had, in his breast pocket, half a dozen pens crammed into a plastic protector. But there's more. He had on horn-rim glasses and hugged a handful of books to his chest like a ten-year-old schoolgirl. Hands down, he was the most pathetic-looking kid in existence.

So what does the dickhead who jumped out of the Jeep do? He goes straight up to the kid, slaps his books out of his hands, and then begins laughing at him and calling him names. Dork, dipshit, fuck nuts—he let this kid have it. Pretty early on in the verbal assault, I suggested that we get moving and, to expedite our departure, started to say that the cops would be showing up. Now, I was certain this short, scrawny kid would begin wailing and running in circles, which only would have prompted this asshole I was with to chase after him.

It would have been a horrible (although hilarious) sight to watch—a two-hundred-and-fifty-pound linebacker chasing down a hundred-and-twenty-pound kid, pens flying everywhere. But that's not what our geek chose to do. Out of nowhere, he charged directly at my dickface associate and swung for the hills.

I couldn't fucking believe it. Swear to God, the football player was so big that even if you had ten buddies getting your back, you'd still think twice about charging him. And here, this little kid was doing it all on his own, petite fists looping through the air like pesky mosquitoes. But before the kid could land a single shot, the football player cracks him and he goes down. I thought that would be it. The kid had probably watched too many kung fu movies and thought he was some kind of tough guy. Daniel-san or some shit. Anyone who saw this exchange would have figured now that he had taken one to the face, he would stay down and play dead. That's not what happened. Getting socked only seemed to fuel his passion for justice. He popped back up like a weeble-wobble and again charged forward.

By this time, another one of the guys in the Jeep had jumped out. Harnessing the pack mentality, he grabbed the kid by his neck, dragged him over to the edge of a grassy slope, and threw him down it. The kid tumbled head over tail, but when he reached the bottom, he didn't lie there in a tattered heap. He came storming back up the hill. When he reached the top, he stopped for a moment, casually removed his glasses, set them down on the grass, and then panned his eyes back and forth between his two assailants. The four words that came hissing out of his mouth will be etched into my frontal lobe for an eternity.

"I'M READY TO DIE!"

He began his charge at five hundred pounds of muscle. He ran straight into one of them and knocked him backward into the Jeep, producing a decent-size dent. This naturally angered the driver, so he jumped out and joined in on the "fun." Together, they began beating the holy hell out of this kid. They'd throw him down, kick him in the guts and back, and then begin to walk away. Before they could make it five feet back to the Jeep, the kid would leap up again and charge them. So they'd smack him around, throw him down again, and do some more kicking. All the while the kid threw his fists for all he was worth, head butting, trying to bite. Meanwhile, I'm urging these boneheads to get moving.

After this went on for a little while, I could see the fear growing in the eyes of my fellow football-player wannabes. They weren't worried about this kid causing them damage with his fists—they were scared of his heart and soul. It suddenly dawned on these geniuses that they had started something they couldn't finish, not unlike a twenty-pound burrito. The kid really was prepared to die for the sake of his dignity. Unless they were willing to go to that end and actually *kill* this kid, they *could not* win this fight. Eventually, the three of them picked the kid up, carried him back to the hill, and threw him over. The second his sinewy frame left their hands, all three of them came scrambling toward the Jeep, scared that they wouldn't make it back before the runt clawed his way up the slope and began his next charge.

All of them fell inside, as though they were trying to escape some terrible onslaught. The driver revved the engine and peeled out. As we sped away from the scene, I looked back over my shoulder. I saw the kid come over the top of the hill in all of his hundred-and-twenty-pound glory, and a chill went down my spine. His face was bloody, and his button-down shirt was torn and grass-stained, but there wasn't a trace of emotion on his face. Instead of running for the police, the kid dusted himself off, put his glasses back on, and then headed casually off, I assume, to Gryffindor or Hogwarts or wherever, hugging his books in his arms. Right then, I realized that not only was that kid the coolest guy in the world, he was the toughest son of a bitch to ever walk the face of this earth.

Toughness can carry you a long way, especially in fighting. Personally, I don't have the best strikes or submissions in the business. The reason I've won most of my fights is that I'm too stupid to back down. It's always been this way. When I was a kid, my mother went to night college, and every afternoon she'd drop me off with a group of older kids. One day when she came to pick me up, she watched them repeatedly chuck me into the bushes. As any mother would do, she stormed over to them and demanded to know what they were doing.

"He's just a little kid!" she shouted.

Immediately they all went on the defensive. "You don't understand. We're playing king of the hill, and he won't quit charging us."

I'm not claiming that those who have a never-say-die attitude are superior to those who don't, because in certain situations, it can actually be detrimental, but when it comes to fighting, it can be one of your most important tools. If an opponent lands fifteen hard punches to your face, and you smile as though you enjoyed the ride, it fucks with his head. After all, the majority of people are equipped with an easily accessible lever in their head that, when pulled, switches them from "fight mode" to "flight mode." We've all seen what flight mode looks like in the Octagon—it can come in the form of severe backpedaling, clinging to your opponent on the ground, or even giving your opponent your arm so he can finish you off with a quick submission. When you take incredible abuse and refuse to make the switch to flight mode, it causes your opponent to doubt that you have the lever in your head at all. At that point, you start to appear more like an angry wild animal than a human. And the majority of us fear angry wild animals because they have no reason. I would have no problem scrapping with a bear or a baboon if I knew that once I hurt it or it hurt me, we'd both say, "Okay, that's enough, time to call it quits and go home." But that's not what angry wild animals do. They don't get into fights; they get into scraps that go to the finish. And once you're lying dead in the dirt, they take it one step further by tearing off your genitals and eating them.

When up against this type of opponent, you don't see the battle as a sport—you see it as a struggle to remain alive, and a lot of fighters aren't prepared for that. It breaks them mentally. A perfect example of a wild animal in the ring is Wanderlei Silva. It doesn't matter how hard or how many times you hit him—as long as his lights are still on, he's coming forward swinging for the fences. The guy fights like a Neanderthal, and that's downright intimidating because in order to stop him, you damn near have to kill him.

The most intriguing fights are when two competitors with this "never back down" attitude square off. A perfect example is when Diego Sanchez fought Karo Parisyan in *UFC Fight Night 6*. Both fighters headed into that battle with the game plan of going balls to wall until the other broke, and they kept that game plan for all three rounds. I got tired just watching them go at it. Another example is my bout with Stephan Bonnar. That fight was fought in both of our heads. For three rounds, it was a nonstop flurry of punches and kicks. The only reason either one of us kept going was that each of us was certain his toughness would break the other. I have since talked with him about that fight, and it was funny because we were both thinking the exact same thing: *I'm catching him with some good shots, and eventually he's going to get tired of this. He's going to break.* However, with both of us being too stupid to quit, neither one of us did.

How do you develop this kind of toughness? The answer is simple—do things that make your body and mind scream at you to quit, but don't (dipshit psychs might call this cognitive behavioral therapy or some bullshit). Personally, I use the treadmill to accomplish this. Every other day, I'll rev that sucker up to twelve miles an hour and do three five-minute intervals. Running at that speed for that duration doesn't come naturally to anyone—it's hideous, absolutely horrible. But by pushing past the pain, you become progressively tougher. You prove to yourself that pain is just that, pain. You can walk away from it afterward knowing that you surpassed a barrier that makes most humans curl into the fetal position and weep for Jesus. If you're not in good shape, you don't have to run at twelve miles an hour. You could run at eight miles an hour, but it is important to set goals for yourself. If eight miles an hour becomes too easy, push it up to nine miles an hour. The most important part is setting a pace that is more than you think you can achieve. It is also important not to do exercises where the pace isn't set. I chose the treadmill over running outside because when I'm on the track, my body naturally slows down as the pain sets in. On a treadmill, you don't have that option.

This mental toughness must be developed BEFORE you start fighting because you don't want to be that guy who quits in the ring—that's unforgivable. Of course, if your opponent has your arm and he gives you a chance to cry uncle before he breaks it, hey brother, you got to tap so you can fight another day. I broke my arm in a fight down in Brazil, and if I'd been given a chance to tap, I would have in a fucking heartbeat. But if you quit because you don't want to get hit anymore, you took the hairy vagina way out. If you want to be a man, take the hits and get knocked the fuck out. My philosophy on getting knocked out is that it renders you unconscious and numb, so why worry about it.

DICK IN A BOX

by Big John

Forrest gave some good advice about how to develop mental toughness, but he failed to mention that in order to develop toughness on an inhuman level, you pretty much have to be insane. He's my best friend, and I want to portray him in a good light, but there is a side to him you don't ever want to see. It's not the crazy, fun-loving side that was captured when he was on *The Ultimate Fighter*—it's the side you see when you piss him off. When I spar with Forrest, I realize he is the better man because he's willing to go places I'm not willing to go. Hell, he'll go places 99.9 percent of human beings are not willing to go. That's why he's been so successful—he can take himself mentally and spiritually to a place where everything is bathed in blood and devilish creatures feed on the limbs of babies. I've heard that Herschel Walker had multiple personality disorder, and although I've taken just a few classes in psychology, I feel safe diagnosing Forrest with the same thing. When he fights or gets angry, he acquires a different personality, and that personality doesn't see limitations or recognize pain.

I'll give you an example. About the time Forrest broke his arm fighting down in Brazil, I had a fellow cop as a roommate. The guy was an absolute tool. He'd introduce himself to chicks as an undercover narcotics agent, and he never shut up. Well, Forrest and me had plans to go out one night, and we brought this guy along to be our designated driver. For hours he went on and on about how much ass he got on the job and how badass he was as a cop. The guy started grating on Forrest in a big way, and when he continued to ramble after we got back to the apartment and began watching a movie, Forrest snapped. Instead of flying off in a rage,

Busting Your Cherry

The first fighting event I ever took part in was a Toughman competition. Did I go through a grueling eight-week training camp to prepare for the show? No, most certainly not. I was a twenty-year-old kid enrolled in the police academy in Athens. I signed up for the event because I had been doing some training with this guy I had met, Robert Fox. He was actually into MMA (or NHB—no

he transformed from the fun-loving Forrest most people know into the sinister one most people don't.

"Could you toss me that lighter?" Forrest asked my douche-bag roommate.

"Sure," the guy said, and tossed him the lighter.

Looking at my roommate straight in the eyes, Forrest positioned the lighter directly underneath his arm and sparked it up. After holding it there for approximately four seconds, he said, "My record is sixteen seconds. Wanna see me break it?"

After another three seconds, the smell of burning flesh filled the room. I couldn't take it anymore, and I knocked the lighter out of his hand. Forrest cracked a smile, and then went back to watching the movie. His arm was a bloody, bubbled mess, but he didn't even treat the wound. I still have no idea why he chose to burn himself, but it served its purpose. My roommate was horrified, and he didn't utter another word for the rest of the night. All he could do was sit there and stare at Forrest. From the look in his eyes, I'm pretty certain he feared for his life.

Now, I've been around awhile, and absorbing that kind of pain isn't normal. Who do you know that can receive a third-degree burn on a substantial part of his body and then just sit there and enjoy a movie? That kind of toughness isn't something you can develop. It originates from lunacy. It might not be a perfect condition if you want to be a refrigerator repairman, but it's tailor-made for fighting. Never once have I been surprised that Forrest has made it as far as he has. The only thing that surprised me was how long it took.

holds barred—as it was called back then—this was '99), but because I had no technique to speak of, we had been taking it one step at a time. At that point, all we had focused on was my boxing. I had a couple of good combinations and a hard punch, but that's it. I entered the event not because I wanted to win the whole thing and begin some fabulous run that would land me in the Toughman Hall of Fame. I simply wanted to sock some people in the face.

DICK IN A BOX

by Luke

White men can't jump, but they can elbow the fuck out of you. If you want to increase your toughness, all you have to do is play basketball Forrest style. I would say that he was a good basketball player, but what he did out there on the court could not rightly be described as basketball. Although he could ali-oop and had a mean crossover, if he got angered by something you did, he would just haul off and try to punch you in the face. This led to several of his more notorious beatings. When he tried to punch Frankie Dickenson in the face for bullying a smaller player, Frankie beat the holy living hell out of him. I've said it before and I'll say it again— never will he get his ass kicked as bad as that day. His face literally got beat in. I remember the coach sentenced them both to cafeteria duty after the fight, and Forrest came in with blood all over him, his face looking like the character Sloth from *Goonies.* Instead of being bummed out like most kids would be, he had a massive smile on his face, as if he had enjoyed the beating. Another time after we had seen the movie *White Men Can't Jump,* we had the bright idea to hustle other kids for money in pickup games. Everything worked out great until we whopped a couple of older kids. They didn't want to pay us, so Forrest got into their grilles. It got a little heated, and suddenly one of them starts punching Forrest in the face as hard as he could. Instead of struggling to get away or fight-

The day of the show I skipped out of the station early, picked Robert up in my piece-of-shit ride, and we made the two-hour drive to Athens, Georgia. The show was being held in the infamous 40-Watt nightclub, which is where R.E.M., the B-52's, and several other popular bands had gotten their start. We walked into the joint, and instead of seeing a bunch of well-conditioned athletes, we were greeted by a host of bikers sporting leather vests and mean-looking tattoos. It looked like a pretty shady competition, and when I caught sight of the ring, it only reinforced that assumption. The promoters of the event had been organized enough to go out and rent an official boxing ring, but apparently their budget was hurting because the ring had failed to come with a bottom

ing back, he just laughed as the guy hit him. It spooked the older kids, and they sprinted away. I still see those guys around town every now and then, and I still ask for our motherfucking money.

I honestly believe that Forrest's involvement in basketball is partially responsible for his toughness today. To develop that toughness, you do not need to be good at basketball or whatever sport you're playing. As a matter of fact, the worse you are, the more likely you'll be to lose your temper or piss off another player. It can sometimes be hard to get into fights when walking down a hall or while hanging out with your friends because you build the fight up in your mind. But when playing a sport such as basketball, your adrenaline is through the roof and you tend to act out your emotions, causing you to start trading blows before you even have a chance to think. And it doesn't have to be basketball. It could be soccer or baseball or even tennis. Forrest played just about every sport our high school had to offer, and he got into fights in all of them. The trick is to play aggressive. I remember one time when Forrest was playing goalie in soccer, a kid was charging toward him with the ball. Instead of focusing on the ball, he focused on the kid and tackled him. While he was on top of him, struggling to make him submit or some shit, the ball rolled casually into the goal. Shortly thereafter, a fight ensued.

rope. Not wanting the fighters to fall out of the ring and onto the toothless women in the front row, they had strung a steel chain where the rope should have been. In case you didn't get that, let me repeat myself. *In place of the bottom rope, they had strung a steel chain.* Now, I'm not a stickler for creating a whole bunch of rules and regulations, but come on. A chain? Really? I suppose barbed wire would have been worse, but not by much. The entire scene was straight out of a Van Damme movie. In hindsight, it was pretty fucking cool.

When it came my time to brawl, I strapped on two eighteen-ounce gloves, both of which were the size of Tito Ortiz's head, and climbed into the ring. I weighed two-forty at the time, and they paired me up with this big fat kid. For the first round we tore into each other with wild, looping punches. We held on longer than the bikers, most of whom gassed after approximately twelve seconds, but by the second round, neither one of us had much left in our tanks. With my wad blown, I drove my opponent back into the ropes so that I could rest my weight on his big fat stomach. Busy sucking in gallon-size gulps of air, he had pretty much given up on trying to hit me. The most I could muster was the occasional body shot.

Now, I'm not sure what this kid was thinking, if he was trying to escape the ring or what, but he stepped one foot over the bottom rope, which as I mentioned was, in fact, a steel chain. At that same moment, I summoned one last ounce of energy and hit him with a good shot that caused him to drop. Somehow his leg got tangled up on the steel chain, and when his weight fell, the chain snapped his tibia in two. Obviously he couldn't continue with a broken leg, so I was declared the winner by technical knockout. Awesome, right?

After I cleaned up, I went looking for this kid to tell him "good fight" or some shit. Instead of finding him on a stretcher getting treated by medical professionals, I found him lying on the pavement out back by the trash cans. I'm not fucking kidding about this—they had dragged this dude out back, dropped him on the greasy pavement by the trash cans, and then left him there. It was as ghetto as you could get, but for some reason the whole experience left me wanting more.

Having won my first bout, I got invited back for the semifinals. Once again, I handled the scrap like any 240-pound dude who was used to winning fights in the street—I went out there and swung for the hills. I gassed just as badly as I had the first time, which is pretty pathetic considering the rounds were only three minutes long, but I did enough to earn another victory. This landed me in the finals, but my championship bout didn't go quite as well. Instead of another roughneck as my opponent, the guy across from me was a fellow student from the University of Georgia. He was longer than me and had a good jab, but every time I got inside on him, I would kill him. The problem was I didn't have the desire to kill him. One time I accidentally stepped on his foot and tripped him up, but instead of capitalizing on his awkward positioning, I let him recover. Another time I had him bent over with his headgear turned around, rendering him blind, but instead of beating his face as though it were a piñata, I backed away so he could straighten it out. The end result is that he got to implement his game plan, which was to utilize his superior reach and pepper me with jabs, and I lost the decision.

When I came back to my corner, Robert looked at me in disgust. "I guess you didn't want to win that one."

"What are you talking about?" I asked.

"You should have hit him. Whenever you have a chance to hit your opponent, you hit him. You don't let opportunities pass you by."

Right then I realized that I had been a nice guy, and nice guys have no business being in the ring. I wanted a rematch. I knew I could beat him the next time around if I fought with my heart and paced myself better, so I kept my eyes open for other Toughman events in the area that he might enter. While on this mission, I got sidetracked by mixed martial arts.

MMA

I was in the grocery store one day, and I ran into this guy I'd seen doing fight training at the Ramsey Physical Education Center at the University of Georgia. We got talking, and he told me that they had an MMA club on campus and that I should come check it out. A couple of days later I picked up a brochure for their club at the phys-ed building, got the times for their classes, and then paid them a visit.

Adam and Rory Singer were sitting on the mats when I walked in, and immediately I liked them. Instead of wearing designer tank tops like a lot of the tampons in the gym, they wore old sweatshirts turned inside out so they wouldn't advertise Bob's Vacuum Repair or whatever gay shit was advertised on the front. They didn't have gel in their hair or smell like they just took a bath in cologne. They looked like dirty mongrels because while in the gym they didn't give a shit about impressing the opposite sex. All they cared about was pumping iron and fighting.

To get my foot in the door, I made up a bunch of lies about my training experience. Those lies were obviously shattered when they mopped the floor with me the first day we did jujitsu, but by that point we had already become friends. So, I started doing jujitsu every Tuesday and Thursday. At first, all we did was gi-training. It wasn't that any of us believed that you had to train with a gi in order to be good at MMA, it's just that Georgia is as humid as a motherfucker, even in the winter. If you tried rolling without pajamas, the mats quickly turned into a slip-and-slide, making submissions impossible. Training with a gi helped add some friction. The only downside was that the uniform would leave scuff marks all over your body. Now that MMA has exploded, explaining the big red welts on your body is as easy as telling people that you grapple, but back in the day people had no idea what grappling was. I would walk into the police academy in the morning with a black eye and red marks all over my neck and face, and my superiors would look at me like I was insane. They all thought I was involved in some type of fight club where the only rules were not to talk about fight club. I remember one time my lieutenant pulled me aside.

"What the fuck is that shit all over your neck?" he asked.

"Oh, it's from my gi," I said. "I was fighting off a choke."

A repulsed look soured his face. "Wait, wait, wait," he said. "You guys carry ropes and try to choke each other? I don't understand—you try to strangle each other with nooses? What kind of things are you into, son? Is it some type of autoerotic asphyxiation?"

I tried to explain it to him further, but he didn't want to listen. I felt like a black sheep, but it didn't stop me from going to jujitsu practice every Tuesday and Thursday. At first I would also go to the Friday class, but it got a little too weird for me. They'd dress up in hockey gear and practice stick fighting. For good measure, they would also throw in a little fake knife fighting. I was interested in neither. When they asked me why I wasn't down, my answer was simple. "I carry a gun, resulting in no need to learn how to fight with a stick or a knife. Just to let you know, I will never engage in fake knife fighting." Ironically, ten years later I'm now getting really into knife fighting and knife throwing. However, I still carry a gun everywhere I go.

For our boxing training, every Monday and Wednesday we'd head over to a gym owned by Donald Kempner. We called him Doc, and despite being one of the world's leading therapists for eating disorders and a multimillionaire, he was one crazy son of a bitch. The stories this guy can tell are endless. I remember one day he came into the gym late, and he said to us, "Hey, if the cops ask, I've been here all day." Sure enough, a short while later the cops roll in and start asking questions.

"Yeah, he's been here," I lied, which was a big deal because I was still going through the academy. "Been in the back, puttering around. What's this about?"

The cops refused to tell me the story, but I got it later from Doc. Apparently, a bicyclist had cut him off while he was driving his car. Instead of letting it go, Doc pulled over. In his passenger seat he always carried two items, a massive tape recorder and a vehicle codebook. The codebook was so he could irritate cops when they pulled him over, and the recorder was to capture the cops saying anything incriminating as a result of his irate ramblings of local ordinance. Angered by the bicyclist, he grabbed the tape recorder, got out of his car, and beat the biker over the head with the device. Not satisfied with the damage he had caused, he threw the bike into the street and drove over it several times. I'm not sure how the scuffle affected him in the long run, but I think that eventually he lost everything after punching one of his patients. A short while after that, he shared his story on *Oprah,* moved to Mexico, and was never heard from again.

After about six months' training with this motley crew, I signed up to compete in an MMA event. It was the same situation as my first Toughman competition—I didn't give a damn about winning or losing, I just wanted to fight. About fifteen minutes before they called me out, I began warming up with a buddy of mine, John Grantham. We started off in the clinch, flowing between light knees and punches, but after a few minutes, we start going harder and harder. I'm getting more and more psyched for the coming bout, and soon we're going full speed. Next thing I know, John lands a brutal knee right to my sternum.

"What the fuck?" I wheezed. Seriously, it felt like he had broken my chest. I got pissed and tried to shove him down, but he was too big to shove anywhere, and that only made me more pissed. While I was still trying to recover from the devastating shot, they called my name. Not willing to back out of a fight for something as minor as a crushed sternum, I made my way to the cage.

The fight wasn't anything to brag about. A few seconds in, I tried to knee my opponent in the head, he fell down, and I fell on top of him. The guy's arm was hanging away from his body, so I locked in an armbar and finished him. My second fight that night went much the same. I moved quickly toward my opponent and tried to kick him in the head, which was strange because I had never trained head kicks. At the time, we only trained in street-fighting techniques, and we had all agreed that kicking to the head wasn't the brightest idea in a street fight. You could lose your balance and fall down or your opponent could catch your leg. Not sure why I did it, but it worked out okay. My opponent fell down, I fell on top of him, and I slapped on another armbar, forcing him to tap.

Did I learn a lot from my Toughman brawls and my first two fights in the cage? I learned that I did pretty much everything wrong. I didn't pace myself properly and, in the case of my MMA fight, got injured a few minutes before being called to the ring (Ken Shamrock would be proud). But you're not meant to get everything right the first time around. If you did, it wouldn't be any fun. The great thing about this sport is that there are so many facets, you always have room for improvement. From my mistakes, I learned that I needed to pace myself better. I also learned that you shouldn't get into a heated sparring session a few minutes before you are supposed to climb in the cage. You're supposed to hit mitts lightly, work on escaping bad positions, and chain stuff together. If the guy who is helping you warm up starts getting rambunctious, you back away from him and find someone else who will help you warm up. These are all things that come with time. However, I was lucky enough to have won my first couple of scraps, which makes staying with the sport all that much easier. For this reason, I recommend not biting off more than you can chew right off the bat. If a promoter is trying to match you up with someone who has twenty fights under his belt, unless he's lost nineteen of them, you'll probably want to find someone who is more on your level. Personally, I recommend fighting someone handicappable. Just don't fight a retarded person. They have retard strength and never give up.

A Beautiful Mind for Fighting

Most intelligent stockbrokers will tell us that the past is not a good indicator of the future, but it's the best indicator we've got. This is especially true in fighting, which makes viewing your opponent's fight tapes extremely important. It can be monotonous and boring, but it is something that both you and your coaches should do before every fight. And you shouldn't watch them like you normally would. You want to analyze them like a mathematician to see patterns. When done properly, it's a lot like buying the cheat guide to a video game—it allows you to see your opponent's strengths and weaknesses before you step into the fight.

The main thing I look for is habits. By watching footage of Quinton Jackson before our fight for the UFC Light Heavyweight title, I picked up on a number of his patterns. His favorite combinations were to throw a left hook and then a right uppercut or a left hook followed by a right hook. I also noticed that he was a very difficult fighter to punch. By keeping his elbows tight to his body and staying relaxed, he had become a master at deflecting fists. In his previous fights, these two habits had worked to his advantage. He'd wait for his opponent to unleash with a combo, block the punches, and then retaliate with one of the aforementioned combinations. With his opponent's guard down as a result of the flurry his opponent just threw, Quinton was routinely able to inflict serious damage with his powerful right hand.

Armed with this knowledge, my coaches and I worked on a game plan. One of my plans was to throw left head kicks at him all night long. Although I knew he would block the majority of them, I wanted to damage his right arm as much as possible to take power away from it. To slow him down on his retaliations and hinder his takedowns, I planned to repeatedly kick him in the legs. And to get past his stellar defense against punches, I planned to throw knees to his body. But watching his tapes helped me most with my movement, I think. Instead of throwing my shots and then standing there in front of him, which would allow him to retaliate, I worked on throwing a combination from one spot and then immediately moving away from it.

As it turned out, I managed to implement a good portion of my game plan. I caught him with a couple good kicks to the leg that decreased his mobility and power, which made it difficult for him to execute his normal speedy retaliations after blocking my combinations. And when he did retaliate, I was able to avoid a lot of his shots because I had worked tirelessly on not standing in one spot. It was a good back-and-forth fight, but in the end, the training I had done to correct my bad habits and capitalize on his allowed me to earn the decision. However, my game plan had not been executed perfectly, and it is important to remember that a fight will never go exactly as you plan. After all, your opponent will most likely have improved from his previous fight. If he's smart, he will have watched your fight tapes and then developed a game plan to capitalize on your weaknesses. In order to win the fight, your game plan has to be stronger than your opponent's. And when I say stronger, I mean the improvements you've made must be more disciplined than the improvements he's made.

All of us have bad habits that we fall back upon in times of stress, and the goal is to force your opponent to retreat to the shelter of his bad habits before he can force you to do it first. For example, let's say you're up against a fighter who has previously had the bad habit of jumping guard (for the five ambitious folks out there reading this book who don't know jujitsu terminology, jumping guard is when you leap into your opponent, wrap your legs around his body, and pull him down on top of you. The purpose of this? You got me.), but he has worked on correcting that mistake for your fight. By staying strong with your game plan and avoiding your own bad habits (the ones he trained to capitalize on), you can frustrate him and force him once again to jump guard. Breaking your opponent in this fashion will usually produce positive results, but the only way to accomplish this is to work on correcting your weaknesses not just in the few weeks leading up to the fight, but over the course of months and years.

What *Not* to Analyze Before a Fight

1) Do not analyze your opponent's cup size because it can be intimidating. For example, Kazushi Sakuraba wears the most gigantic cup known to man. Am I the only one who has noticed this? He's got to do it as a mind-fuck, kind of like how the U.S. Army dropped huge condoms on Vietnam so the Asian guys would be intimidated by our cock sizes. And it does work to an extent. Stare at Sakuraba's cup for long enough, it's downright scary.

2) Do not analyze your opponent's prefight rituals. For example, Rashad Evans has been known to repeatedly twist his nipples before his fights. That seems problematic to me. It worries me.

Wash Your Balls

I'm going to veer off course for a moment, but this is important . . . If you haven't washed your balls in four days and your feet smell like you've soaked them for half an hour in a bucket of dog shit, please, please do not come to grappling practice. I'm serious—don't even leave the house. There is nothing worse in this world than rolling around on the mats with a guy who reeks like Rosie O'Donnell's greasy butt crack. If you've grappled for a couple of years at a number of different places, you know exactly what I'm talking about. You know exactly *whom* I'm talking about. When you close your eyes, you can still see the silhouette of that gangly kid with pee-stained board shorts, his rankness flowing on a river of sweat into your ears and other orifices. Forgive me for being insensitive, ladies, but I imagine it's a lot like being sexually assaulted; after the fact, you drive home with a faraway look in your eyes and then suddenly wake up in the shower, your skin raw from having scrubbed yourself down with a wire brush. It's a harrowing experience many of us never recover from, so I have no remorse for the assailants in these dastardly acts. If you happen to be a swamp creature that has no respect for yourself or those you come into contact with, do not take a shower and wash your clothes. It is too late for that—you've already ruined lives. Simply find the nearest solid object and repeatedly run your face into it until you cease to exist. You're a walking, talking fungal factory, and you have no right being here.

The reason I sound a bit harsh is that I've been victimized by general filthiness on multiple occasions. In one such assault, I received a nasty staph infection. I'm not going to give you the clinical definition (too lazy to look that shit up), but all you really need to know is that it fucking sucks. The worst part is that it's easy to miss. If an area of your skin is infected, it will become red, swollen, and painful, but when you grapple on a regular basis, all sorts of chaffing occurs. It can be difficult to distinguish between regular wear and tear and a gross staph infection that, if gone untreated, can have all sorts of horrible consequences, including paralysis or death. Because I turned my body into a punching bag, that's what happened to me. I picked up a healthy case of staph from some slimy douche bag, didn't realize it, and then went to Georgia to get some training in at the Hardcore Gym. The first day we did wind sprints, which I'm normally quite good at, and everyone in the place killed me. I was as fatigued as a midget actor at an Ewok convention. I thought that perhaps I had picked up the flu on the plane and decided to wait it out, but I kept feeling weaker and weaker. Eventually, I went to a Quick Care in Athens. Apparently, doctors at walk-in clinics can't tell the difference between a staph infection and an asshole, because he gave me antibiotics for a sinus infection and sent me on my way. I was told to wait it out, which I attempted to do. A few days later, I literally thought I was going to die.

I flew back to Vegas and saw a real doctor. By this time, an irritated patch of redness had materialized on my knee. The doctor identified it as staph, squeezed out some pus, and then wrote me a prescription for an antibiotic. I was more than relieved to have found the source of my misery because I had an upcoming bout against Lyoto Machida over in England. I needed to get my ass back to the gym, but that didn't end up happening. Despite popping the pills I was given, I continued to get worse. When the pain and overall horribleness became unbearable, I went to see a different doctor. He ran some tests, and it was determined that I had staph in my blood. Fucking great. I ended up being on antibiotics for five weeks and, as a result, I had to back out of the fight against Machida.

I apologize about this rather long-winded story, but hopefully I have struck the fear of God into you. Staph infections suck, as do all the other bacteria and funguses that you can pick up from foul wrestling mats and unclean people. To limit your risk, it is important to make sure the mats in your gym are clean. Approaching the owner of the gym and asking him about the process he uses to clean the mats might make you look like an anal asshole (no, that's not redundant—I'm talking about the other kind of anal dumbshit), but it's better than hoping for the best and ending up with a mat-born disease. If he says something like, "You got to clean the mats? Really?", pass this information on to him:

1) **Wrestling mats should be cleaned twice daily with disinfectant cleaner, and this should be done two hours before each grappling session. For the best results, you want to use one cup of bleach for every hundred cups of water.**

2) **Street shoes should not be allowed on the wrestling mats. Dogs and other animals carry all sorts of bacteria, and they shit and roll around everywhere. If you step in a puddle of their filth and then walk on the mats, you might very well be giving all your training partners the gift of ringworm.**

3) **All gym equipment such as boxing gloves, shin pads, belly pro-
   tectors, and headgear should be routinely sprayed with disinfectant.**

Training at a gym that maintains a clean environment will certainly lessen your chances of picking something up, but it's still not a guarantee. If there is an outbreak of some type of bacteria or fungus among your training partners, you need to be cautious. I once saw an episode of *The X-Files* where Mulder and Scully stripped naked and checked each other for infection. Although you probably don't want to take it to this extreme because it will make your training partners uncomfortable, especially if you attempt to examine them in the shower, it can't hurt to give their upper body a "once-over" just to be on the safe side. Below, I give brief descriptions of some of the bacterial and fungal infections to look out for:

Ringworm

Contrary to popular belief, ringworm is not actually a worm. It's a disease caused by a fungus. To spot it, look for a patch of rough, reddened skin that is hard in the center and spans outward. If the wound looks like it was created by worms, it's probably ringworm. There are many types of ringworm—body ringworm, scalp ringworm, ringworm of the nails, and ringworm of the groin (although I've never personally had this one, I imagine that it would really, really suck). The majority of the time, ringworm is transmitted from skin-on-skin contact. Sometimes the disease will go away on its own, but most cases should be treated with medication.

Staphylococcal Infection (Staph)

When you get a staph infection, pus-filled pockets will usually pop up just beneath the skin. If gone untreated, these pockets will eventually grow so bloated that they explode, dribbling pus onto other areas of your body and causing new infection. It is also possible for staph to enter your bloodstream and spread throughout your body, which is what happened to me. This is known as an invasive staph infection, and it can do nasty stuff to your lungs, kidneys, brain, and heart. If you suspect you have a staph infection, you should go to the doctor immediately and get treated.

Impetigo

There are two types of impetigo, and both are highly contagious. The first is called bullous, and it appears as a large bump on the skin that has a tip filled with clear fluid. It usually won't become painful or red, but it will probably itch like a mother. The other kind of impetigo, called epidemic, will also appear as a small bubble of liquid, but surrounding the sac will be a red ring. Both types are usually easily cured with antibiotics, but if left unchecked, they can lead to serious diseases, such as bone infection.

Herpes

We all know that herpes is the gift that keeps on giving. What many people don't know, however, is that it's not just transmitted by engaging in dirty deeds with filthy whore bags. As far as skin diseases transmitted through wrestling or grappling, it's right up there on the list. When a carrier has an outbreak, they will get small bumps that quickly transform into fluid-filled blisters. The virus is usually passed on through skin-on-skin contact. Although carriers are most contagious during an outbreak, they can also pass on the virus during times of remission. There is currently no way to cure herpes, but there are antiviral drugs that can lessen the duration of outbreaks.

Scabies

Scabies is particularly disgusting because it is caused by tiny little insects called "mites." There are male and female mites, but the males are cool. Just as with everything, the females cause all the problems. When experiencing PMS, they will burrow underneath your skin and lay their eggs. After a short time, the eggs hatch and a host of mite babies surface. Being horny creatures, they don't go on dates or engage in foreplay—they immediately begin mating with one another (incestuous little bitches) and lay more eggs in the skin of the host or any unlucky person the host decided to grapple with that day. Unlike many skin infections, scabies can sometimes be difficult to spot. You want to look for slightly raised gray lines on the skin—the path mites burrow. The primary symptom is an irritating itchiness, which is caused by an adverse reaction to the insects' feces. Scratching is promoted because it will often remove the little buggers from their incestuous love dens, but please do not do this while lying in your training partner's guard. If scratching doesn't do the trick, your doctor will most likely prescribe some type of lotion. Lube those babies up, and you should be ready to go.

Grappling Partners to Avoid

People Who Have No Sphincter Control

Everyone on this planet blows ass every now and then. I blow ass, you blow ass, and that superhot chick with a rockin' body blows superstinky ass from time to time. However, the majority of us can somewhat control when we blow ass and when we don't. If I step into a crowded elevator, I most likely won't blow ass. I'll wait until I'm just about to get off to let the gust of foulness seep out of my body. Back in the day, when I first met a chick, there was no way I would let one rip. I would wait until at least the second or third date before I introduced her to my Love Potion 109. You see what I'm getting at here—by simply clenching up on the vault doors, you can hold those toxins in. And if there ever was a time to hold in a fart, it's when you're grappling at the gym. I understand that sometimes emergencies happen, but usually you see those emergencies coming and have the common courtesy to let go of your submission and walk across the room before letting one fly. But there are guys who have no fart control to speak of. These are the types of guys who will not just fart around you, but also fart on you. Neil Melanson, a grappling coach at Xtreme Couture, has one such horror story. On this fateful day, he was drilling with his student Crazy Jimmy in the north-south position. If you're unfamiliar with this position, it's where the guy on top has got his ass directly on top of his opponent's face. In this unfortunate situation, Neil happened to be the guy on the bottom. He was just lying there, allowing his student to work his submissions, and then Jimmy farted horribly. Traveling directly from ass to mouth, the noxious gas didn't have a chance to get diluted by pure air. Neil literally ate shit. He has not yet recovered from this experience, and to this day he is still in counseling. In my opinion, there is no excuse for this. The majority of us were born with sphincter muscles, and it is our obligation to learn how to use them. If someone in your gym has failed to acquire this courteous training, do not grapple with him under any circumstance.

Extreme Sweaters

If at all possible, try to avoid grappling with people who sweat profusely. I realize that it is no fault of their own, but it is gross. When they're on top, their sweat will often puddle in your ears, drip into your mouth and nose, and make you feel utterly nasty in every way possible.

Marathon Grapplers

There are a lot of guys who will go to two or three grappling classes in a row, but for some reason they think it unimportant to bring a fresh T-shirt for each class. Although you will most likely end up sweaty halfway through practice, it is horribly jarring to walk into the gym fresh and begin grappling with a guy with clammy skin and a sweat-soaked shirt. Seriously, it's like grappling with a fish.

Claw Boy

Claw boy is the kid who sees no reason to trim his fingernails or toenails before practice. If you've never grappled, you might think it a trivial thing to bitch about, especially given the brutal nature of MMA. But trust me, a guy with unkempt nails is essentially armed with twenty miniature daggers. Five minutes of grappling with one of these douche bags can turn you into a bloody mess. You end up with foot-long scrape marks across your thighs and, more commonly, the back of your neck. To prevent leaving the gym looking like you just escaped a Vietnam prison camp, always carry a set of clippers with you to practice.

Shadow Man

Men usually shave first thing in the morning, and jujitsu practice tends to be in the evenings. If you're one of those men who grow facial hair at an alarming rate, please shave again before coming to practice. Beards are totally cool, but rolling with someone who has a five-o'clock shadow sucks. Seriously, that quarter centimeter of stubble you think looks so cool is essentially sandpaper, and it has the ability to shave skin off your opponent's body. If you've got one of these Don Johnson–type douche bags in your gym, avoid him like the plague until he mows his face.

The Band-Aid King

Band-Aids can be found in every medicine cabinet and people love them. They can be used to hide nasty pimples from the world or prevent cuts and scrapes from getting infected. In the everyday world, people who use Band-Aids are smart. In the grappling world, people who use Band-Aids are seriously retarded. I understand them wanting to prevent an open wound from smearing in their opponent's face, but they must have experienced some serious head trauma to actually believe that the minor adhesive holding the Band-Aid in place can endure a heated grappling match. Unfortunately, the majority of the time the Band-Aid doesn't simply fall off—it transfers from his skin to yours. Sometimes you are completely unaware of this transference until you get home and your girlfriend looks at you funny and says, "I think you have something stuck to your neck." She peels it off, and sure enough, you find your training partner's bloody Band-Aid that mysteriously vanished during training. To avoid this outcome, cover all wounds with the tape you use to wrap your hands.

Warthogs

You should avoid grappling with guys who have excessive warts for the same reasons you should avoid grappling with guys who wear Band-Aids—they get torn off and end up stuck to the side of your face.

A Good Heart Ain't Just a Punchy Metaphor for Toughness

If you want to improve your conditioning for fighting, you must do sports-specific cardio workouts. Running and plyometrics are both great, but they should be seen as icing on the cake. Personally, I design my workout to resemble a pyramid (similar to the tried-and-true Food Pyramid), the base of which is live sparring. For example, I'll do position sparring where I'm on my back for three one-minute rounds. In each round, a fresh fighter comes in and takes the top position. It works out great for him because he is fresh and can go balls out for his one minute, practicing his ground-and-pound, going for submissions, and working his passes. And it works out great for the guy on bottom because he has to suffer and survive for three rounds with fresh fighters. Not only is this key for developing your stamina, but it also teaches you how to relax. Floyd Mayweather Jr. has hands like lightning because he always remains calm and relaxed. When he moves, he is resting, and as a result he never gets tired. It's the same with Anderson Silva.

It is also important to break down why you are doing something. For example, at the beginning of practice I'll often hit mitts. My goal is not to develop cardio, but rather to work on form and speed. So I'll make sure every punch I throw is perfect and crisp. I keep my hands up, and utilize exact and deliberate movements. Then, at the end of the day, I'll go back to the mitts, but this time, instead of working to improve my form, I work for conditioning. I still keep my hands up and chin down, but since now my intentions are different, my punches don't have to be perfect. I'll go past the point of exhaustion to simulate how the fight will truly be. If I have anything left over, I go running. As Wanderlei says, "It's better to push yourself in training than in the weight room." After all, you're not going to try to deadlift your opponent or bench-press your way out of a rear-naked choke. Chances are you'll spend a lot more time punching and grappling with an opponent, and so that is how you should get your cardio— through punching and grappling. I have a friend who constantly does plyos, jumps rope, and runs three miles in nineteen minutes. When he got totally gassed out in a fight, he asked me why. My answer was simple: "You hardly ever spar, stupid."

I'm not saying that you shouldn't go running, because it can be very beneficial for strengthening your lungs and toughening up your body. I'm just saying that you should go running after you have already gotten your sports-specific training out of the way.

Thou Shalt Spread
Thy Seed Before Weigh-ins

You may have picked up this book simply to read my thoughts on sex before a fight, and I think that's disgusting. But since you're already reading, I suppose I should give you my thoughts, under the assumption that you're reading this book for the sake of sharpening your fighting-dar and not for the visual of me getting my prefight on.

I think you *absolutely* should have sex the night before the weigh-ins. Go ahead and shed a little bit of that nervous energy and sweat a little. At the very least, you'll lose a pound or two—which could make the difference between a big payday and humiliation, fat ass. But with regard to prepugilistic sex, think of it this way: sex gets your heart going, and anything that gets your heart going is good for fighting. To be entirely honest, not that you asked (but I know you're thinking it, perv), I hardly ever have sex before a fight, but it's not because I think it will somehow drain my chi. Usually, I'm just so overtrained that I'm too banged up to bang. I simply can't get it up. But if you do have sex, don't have crazy sex. If you're with a new chick, you'll obviously want to make a time of it, get a little rough. You have to be careful with this—if you're going full board and can last for more than five minutes, you're liable to get penis chaffing, which will get aggravated tenfold in your cup while fighting. The risk obviously lessens when you're actually able to make the woman wet, but come on, who really worries about that.

When pounding away like a construction worker, it's also possible to get physically injured. This can happen when your erection has an unfortunate, high-impact collision with your chick's pelvic bone, causing your schlong to forcibly fold in one direction or another. The blood vessels inside the shaft rupture, leading to what is often referred to as "Broke Dick." The best way to avoid this injury prior to your fight is to politely ask your lady to blow you (and, for the lady fighters—you know who you are—ask politely for your guy to, um, do the deed and go downtown). If she really cares about you, she'll do it without hesitation. No one gets hurt, and no one goes away unhappy. So have no fear about getting some, just don't go boogie nights with it.

Sweep the Leg

If you've ever seen the movie *The Karate Kid*, you undoubtedly remember the final fight scene between Daniel-san and evil Johnny from the even eviler Cobra Kai dojo. It was the ultimate battle between good and evil—the most intense fight scene ever captured on film. The Karate Kid is limping around the point-sparring mats, one knee jacked up beyond belief. Johnny is all fired up, his sleeveless black gi covered in point-sparring sweat. All the mothers in the crowd call the name of their hero, creating a ravenous roar for blood that could

DICK IN A BOX

by Luke

Things You Might Not Want to Know About Forrest

1) As a child, Forrest had an insatiable desire for a pair of black leather pants.

2) In high school we'd sometimes play the drinking game "quarters." When it was Forrest's turn to drink, he would consume not only the beer, but also the quarter at the bottom of the cup. In one game, he swallowed a buck fifty.

3) When Forrest went to court for a street fight in high school, the judge asked him if he had anything to say. Forrest replied, "Yeah, I have something to say, but I don't want it to be used against me." The judge shook his head and returned, "Son, you're in court. Everything will be held against you."

4) In high school, Forrest's favorite basketball team was the Spurs, and his favorite player was Dennis Rodman. Although he doesn't have any tattoos, he has always admired hustlers and people who have no problem being themselves.

5) Forrest is good friends with most of the people who kicked his ass in high school.

6) Forrest accidentally brought a loaded gun through an airport X-ray machine. He was arrested, but the charges were later dropped.

7) Forrest has the bad habit of constantly grabbing and fondling his pecker. In high school, chicks would always come up to me and say,

have stifled the cries of the heathens that filled the stands of the Colosseum in ancient Rome. Who is going to win this epic battle? It is close—too close. Before the fighters step to each other for the final exchange of slaps, Johnny's sensei pulls him aside and utters those three infamous words, *SWEEP THE LEG.* Like an ancient sun trying to peer over the horizon of a darkened land, Johnny's rough exterior breaks for a moment, showing the flame of compassion rising up

"We think your friend Forrest is cute and everything, but why is he always grabbing his dick?" Forrest's defense is that he had hernia surgery, and he wants to check to make sure everything is still there.

8) In middle school, Forrest was obsessed about people thinking he was gay. Normally, when two guys go to the movies, they'll leave one seat between them. This is commonly referred to as the "gay seat." Forrest insisted on a "gay aisle." He'd shout over at me, "Hey, do you think people will think we're gay?" I'd reply, "I'm pretty sure people won't think we even know each other."

9) If Forrest is passed out and you pour beer on his face, he will wake up and put you in a triangle hold until you pass out. Fact.

10) In high school, Forrest had sex with his girlfriend in the front row of a Lords of Acid concert.

11) When Forrest encounters two guys fighting in the street, he will immediately break them apart. Instead of sending them on their way, he'll give them a quick coaching lessen and then referee the bout.

12) Forrest's middle name is Estergall, but he recently paid forty-five dollars to have it legally changed.

13) Forrest and I used to train and spar drunk all the time. We figured that if we were to get into a street fight, we'd most likely be drunk, and we wanted to be prepared.

from the most distant recesses of his being, but that compassion wanes as quickly as it has waxed, and then the grasp his dastardly instructor has over his conscious mind once again takes hold. *Yes,* Johnny thinks, a sinister gleam in his eye. *Yes, I am going to sweep Daniel-san's bad leg. I'm going to attack his weaknesses and then bathe in his innards!*

I know what you're thinking: *Forrest, you fucked that all up. It was WAY more intense than that.* Yes, I know. But I had to re-create the scene because I have a question for you. In your opinion, do you think the evil sensei was wrong to tell Johnny to sweep Daniel-san's leg? If you think it was disgusting advice, that he should have instead told his student to ignore the leg and try to win by attacking Daniel-san's strengths, consider yourself a martial artist. If you feel his instruction was spot on, that perhaps he should have added "break that wounded pipe cleaner in half and put that Miyagi wannabe down for good," then, and *only* then, can you consider yourself a fighter.

If you're sitting there right now, nodding your head and thinking, *Yep, I'm a martial artist, and proud to be one,* you know absolutely nothing about fighting. You think you know something about fighting, but you don't. Chances are you're a fat, middle-aged man who wears pajamas and runs his mouth at least twice a week about the effectiveness of dim mak and how you could kill any MMA fighter with a single touch. I'm not trying to insult you. If your delusion makes you happy, more power to you. I'm just trying to clarify the difference between fighters and most martial artists. For the record, fighters are people who actually compete in real fights. Their sparring gear isn't constructed from cheap plastic a quarter of an inch thick because they actually hit one another. They do not throw punches from the hip because they realize the practicality of protecting their face. They know if the techniques shown to them really work because they test them every day in the gym and in the ring. They've beaten the shit out of people and had the shit beaten out of them, and through such beatings they've not only become mentally and physically tough, but have also learned that fighting is a dog-eat-dog world. If your opponent's leg is injured and it floats away from his body, you latch onto that sucker and go for the submission. He has the option to tap, but if he's too late or too stupid, it's really not your fault. You don't want to *try* to break your opponent's leg, but what happens, happens. Going easy to avoid injuring your opponent is a good way to get your ass kicked.

In my experience, people involved in MMA call themselves fighters. People who talk about fighting call themselves martial artists. But then again, GSP calls himself a martial artist . . . In order not to screw up my theory, I think he should gain a bunch of weight, lose his good looks, and take up point sparring. That's all I have to say about that.

Finish Him!

If you want to be a good grappler, play as many video games as possible. Personally, I suck at video games, which is the reason my jujitsu isn't off-the-charts good. Jeremy Horn, Mike Pyle—all the guys who have sick jujitsu play an obscene amount of video games. It helps with your eye/hand coordination or some shit like that. As a matter of fact, I think Mark Lamen actually has his students play video games to get better at jujitsu.

Cutting Weight One Pound at a Time
(or, Kill the Siamese Sumo, Chunky Trunks)

Although weight cutting can be a brutal experience, it is a vital activity in the fight game—you don't make weight, you don't fight. As a rule of thumb, you want to compete in the weight class below your natural weight. If you weigh 170 pounds, you want to compete in the 155-pound division. If you walk around at 220 pounds like me, you want to compete at 205 pounds in the light heavyweight division. The goal is to drop weight the night before the event for the weigh-ins, and then quickly put the weight back so you have a weight advantage over your opponent. Every fighter has a different method for shedding the extra pounds before a fight. It's impossible to say which one is best because everyone handles weight loss differently. The important part is finding a method that works for you. To help steer you in this direction, I'll give you my personal strategy.

I start cutting a week before the fight. For a Friday weigh-in, I'll progressively taper my food intake down on Monday and Tuesday. Wednesday I start the hard-core dieting. Instead of eating meals, I'll snack just enough throughout the day to keep my body standing upright. The majority of my caloric intake consists of oatmeal and other healthy foods. To flush my body out, I'll drink around three gallons of distilled water. During the day on Thursday, I do the exact same thing—snack here and there and consume approximately three gallons of distilled water. Come Thursday night, I'll throw on the plastics and run, jump rope, and do a light workout on the focus mitts. My goal is to get within ten pounds of my fighting weight. A lot of fighters will try to drop all of the extra weight the night before, but then you have to maintain that weight for the next twenty-four hours, which can zap your energy and make you sick. Other fighters will leave more weight to cut the following day, but when you try to cut more than ten pounds at the last minute, you can hurt yourself. For me, ten pounds is the happy medium. The important part is not to stress. If you're within ten pounds, the weight will come off. When I go to sleep, I'll bring a small bottle of water with me to wet my lips, but for the most part, water is out.

Friday morning I'll get up and shed the last few pounds by throwing on the plastics and walking and running on the treadmill. If that doesn't do the trick, I'll keep the plastics on and lie down to sweat in my sleep.

Once you make weight, it is very important to rehydrate yourself. I like to mix Pedialyte with regular water, not distilled. Just make sure you don't drink beverages with high quantities of sugar or potassium because you'll likely shit yourself in the ring. I would give you advice on what to do if you do happen to shit yourself in the ring, but thankfully this has not happened to me yet. I heard it happened to Tim Sylvia while fighting Assuerio Silva and to Kevin Randleman when fighting Renato Sobral. They might be able to give you some better advice; but I would think that if the fight wasn't stopped, this could give one an advantage—I can't imagine that a triangle choke, sunk in by a fellow with turd-soaked trunks, would be too pleasant for the recipient. It may be more important to find out the other side's answer, what to do if you find yourself being the Shitee. Yeah, that might actually be more important.

In addition to rehydrating yourself, you also want to pack your weight back on. Personally, my goal is to get back up to my normal weight of 220 pounds, and I accomplish this by eating sweet potatoes, wheat bread, and some easily digestible chicken. You want to stay away from superheavy food that is hard to digest, like burgers and fries. You made it this far, what's one more day?

The day of the fight you most likely won't have much of an appetite, but it is important to eat some healthy food when you wake up, such as eggs, oatmeal, or some more of those damnable sweet potatoes. Although you want to stay heavy, you don't want to overeat. When I fought Elvis Sinosic, I had a lot of weight to cut, and I took it off fairly easily. But I felt like utter shit afterward. I was weak and exhausted, and in an attempt to turn that feeling around and put the weight back on, I'd eat until I was sick and lie down. When I had enough energy to get back up, I'd go eat more. I managed to recoup my strength and even shoot up to 224 pounds, but there was a side effect. I went into the fight feeling like there was a cannonball in my stomach. Swear to God, I felt as if there were goldfish swimming around in there. I would have been better off stepping into the fight light.

Another time when my weight cutting went terribly wrong was when I fought Hector Ramirez over in Ireland. I showed up three days before weigh-ins, and I weighed 226 pounds. Normally that would have been no sweat to cut (no pun intended—that's just my comedic genius), but in Ireland they didn't have distilled water. Also, all their foods were drenched in grease. If I ordered egg whites, they'd drench them in oil. If I ordered oatmeal, they'd give me this mashed stuff with sweet cream already in it. Delicious, but not a part of any diet I've heard of. If I had ordered a salad, I'm sure they would have soaked it for half an hour in a bucket of bacon grease. So when you cut weight, take context into account, as well as the little add-ons. Lettuce don't automatically make something healthy, dipshit.

If you're not sure about how a certain weight-cutting diet will work for you, I recommend testing it out three or four months before a fight. If you still have your doubts, diet to be on the light side. With fans having paid their hard-earned buck to see you compete, the last thing you want to do is come in over.

Wanna Go Pro? Start Packing

A lot of people will tell you to travel to different gyms and train with as many fighters as possible, and I agree with this to a certain extent. It's always beneficial to train with a new set of guys and learn new ideas. Although I'm based out of Vegas, I've traveled to train at AKA in California. However, once fighting has become your career, this is much harder to manage. When I go on the road now, I don't have my strength coach, I don't have my routine, I don't have all the guys who are working for me to prepare me for my next fight. And, after getting fucked up by the fatty foods over in Ireland—which made it more difficult for me to make weight—I don't even like traveling to fight. Too many, um, distractions. For me, the negatives just aren't worth the rewards. Fighters like Randy Couture and Chuck Liddell, both of whom practically *live* on the road, can do it just fine, but they've both been in the business for more than a decade and are much more manly than me. My advice is that instead of traveling to train, you should move

DICK IN A BOX

by Adam Singer

**Advice for the Fat and *Tremendously* Out-of-Shape Fighter
Who Has No Business Being in the Cage**

There are a lot of guys out there who want all the glory that goes along with being a fighter, but they're too lazy to put in the hard work. If you happen to fall into this category, following the tips below will allow you to survive and possibly even triumph in the cage.

1) Appearance is everything. A bald head and goatee will do wonders to intimidate your opponent. Add a tribal tattoo into the mix, and you're pretty much guaranteed a victory.

2) Block all punches with your forehead. Getting hit in the face really hurts and it screws up your appearance. Your head is much harder than your face.

3) Throw nonstop overhand rights with your eyes closed. It's not important to know where your punches are heading or even look at your target. Just swing for the fences. If you hit the referee, tell him that it was his fault for not getting out of the fucking way.

to a city where the training is prevalent, places like Los Angeles, San Diego, or Las Vegas. In Vegas, a ten-minute drive will take you to five different gyms. It's the best of both worlds—you get to maintain your daily routine, yet still get introduced to new people and ideas. If you're unwilling to move away from your hometown or leave your current job for the sake of getting the training you need, you should probably make MMA your hobby rather than your profession. Unfortunately, fighting takes commitment on all levels, plain and simple.

A Profound Word on Nutrition

Never scramble a can of tuna with egg whites because it will make your entire house smell like dead fish for at least a month. Your cats go crazy, your friends

4) Steroids, steroids, steroids. This magic elixir can replace all forms of training and will add to your intimidating appearance.

5) Only fight in your hometown. Why? Your fans will cheer loudly enough that even a smart referee will think you won the fight. If the referees ignore the crowd's zeal and rule for your opponent, you still may get a decent-size riot out of it.

6) If all of the above tips fail, curl into the fetal position and beg for mercy.

7) After the fight, instead of getting treated by the doctor backstage, walk around the crowd making excuses. To get the best response from the chicks, you should be wearing your fight trunks, have no shirt on, and still be covered in your own blood. A few weeks later, tell everyone you're a UFC fighter.

8) Forrest and Big John used to train and spar drunk all the time. They figured that if they were to get into a street fight, they'd most likely be drunk, and they wanted to be prepared.

give you funny looks when they come over, and your girlfriend will be pissed. It's just not a good idea.

The Cage Is Your Home. You Too Good for Your Home?

If you want to compete in mixed martial arts, it's obvious that you need to develop fighting skills that you can use in the cage, but what's less obvious and *almost* as important is to learn how to use the cage to increase your fighting ability.

The first thing you must learn is how to maintain your bearings. Unlike square rings, the majority of cages are circular, making it easy to lose track of where you are. Instead of glancing at the surrounding chain link, which can sometimes be difficult to focus on, I'll pay attention to the black line painted on the canvas a few feet in from the fence. If I'm facing the center of the cage and the line is directly underneath my feet, I know that the fence is right behind me. If I'm facing the center of the cage and the line is underneath my opponent's feet, I know his back is near the fence. This is valuable information because the cage can work for you or against you.

When your back is up against the fence, one of your escape routes has been lost, making you more vulnerable to your opponent's attacks. If your opponent's back is up against the fence, he is vulnerable to your attacks. As a result, the goal in any fight is to cut angles using footwork to force your opponent to step to the outside of that black line. This might sound easy, but it's often very difficult. To be effective, you must anticipate where your opponent wants to move and then move into that location before he does. When done properly, you can pretty easily steer him around the cage.

Once you have your opponent backed up against the chain link, it can be difficult to keep him confined in one spot because of the lack of sharp corners, so it is important to seize the moment and either launch a combination or tie him up in the clinch and pin his back to the fence. If you choose the latter option, you have all sorts of offensive maneuvers at your disposal, such as dropping down to seize his legs or throwing close-range striking combinations. Because of his inability to retreat backward, your techniques will be more effective and powerful.

The cage can also be used to your advantage when on the ground. When you're in the top position, dragging your opponent over to the perimeter of the cage and then pinning his head up against the chain link allows you to seriously limit his mobility. Many, many fights were won this way in the early days, but in recent years fighters trapped on the bottom have become masters at walking their back up the fence to escape back to their feet. It is important to learn this technique, but you must be careful with it. When I used this walk-up technique in my fight with Hector Ramirez, he punched me in the side of my face, causing my ear to poke through the chain link on my way up. It hurt like a sumofabitz. So here's a tip—don't have big ears if you can help it.

In addition to learning offensive maneuvers for when you push your opponent back into the fence, you must also learn defensive maneuvers for when he drives your back into the cage wall. The goal is to dive your arms underneath his arms before he can do the same to you. If you fail and he secures double underhooks, clasping his hands together behind your back will give him a body lock, which allows him to do all sorts of nasty stuff, such as picking you up and dropping you on your head. It's obviously best to avoid this lock altogether, but is important to always be prepared for the worst-case scenario.

When my back is up against the fence and my opponent secures a body lock, I'll use a technique that Tito Ortiz showed to my old coach, Rory Singer. It's called the back scratch because that's exactly what you do—rub your back up and down the chain link. With your opponent's hands clasped together in the small of your back, his knuckles grate painfully on the steel mesh, causing him to release his hold. If this doesn't work and he picks you up to execute a takedown, you have a couple of options: 1) Allow him to succeed and then either work back to your feet using the cage wall or attempt to reverse your positioning using a sweep. 2) Grab onto the fence to prevent him from accomplishing his goal. Grabbing the fence is illegal in MMA, but if you know you have no chance of surviving if the fight gets brought to the ground, sometimes it's your best option. The referee will often take a point away for breaking the rules, which is what happened when Tito grabbed the fence to prevent Rashad Evans from taking him down. When asked about the tactic after the fight, Tito said, "If you ain't cheating, you ain't trying." I would have to agree with him. I would rather be known as a cheater than a loser. Seriously, I have this deep hatred for losing. If someone were to give me the option of failing at something or having my nuts crushed with a hammer, I would probably take the hammer . . . And yes, I did just say I'd do what Tito Ortiz did.

Back to Basics
(or, Save the Flashy Moves for Your Eighties Prom, Shabba Doo)

For a couple of years I was working out with a personal trainer, and he had me doing all the hip new exercise regimens, such as core training, kettle bells, and resistance training with rubber bands. Although I got something from each workout, I came to the conclusion that too much of any one gimmick is not good. Most of the time, you'll benefit a lot more by focusing on the basics. It's okay to supplement the basics with kettle bells or band training, but you definitely want to develop your base through good old-fashioned lifting. It's the same with fighting. Developing a mean spinning head kick and other flashy moves can certainly add to your fighting prowess, but you probably won't get anywhere in fighting if that's all you have in your arsenal. If you were forced to choose between flashy techniques and basic ones, always choose the basic ones. A good right cross will carry you a lot further in the Octagon than a crescent kick, just as a strong understanding of basic positioning will take you a lot further on the ground than a bunch of fancy submissions. Once you develop a strong foundation based on the basics, it's okay to add some slick moves to your game. Just don't base your game on those slick Bruce Lee moves.

Repeat After Me: I Am Invincible

When your opponent lands a hard punch to your face, do not shake your head in an attempt to clear the fuzziness away. This isn't baseball and there is no pitch count. I don't care how many bells are going off in your skull, shaking your head only tells your opponent "I'm hurt—please come hit me again." You also don't want to nod your head, which is a bad habit a lot of fighters pick up in the gym when sparring with friends. I used to do this all the time, but it only gives your opponent positive reinforcement. I don't care how badly you're hurt, you never want to give any tells. A perfect example of a guy who shows nothing in the ring is Wanderlei Silva (despite what you're thinking, I don't have a hard-on for Wandy—okay, okay, maybe I do). You could run the guy over with a dump truck, and he would pop back up and be like, "What, that's all you got? Fucking pussy." Fedor's facial expressions are even better because it looks like he doesn't even know he is in a fight.

"Rudy, Rudy . . ."

From inside the cage, there are two ways to win the crowd. The first way is to be one of the best fighters on the planet. I'm not talking about a good fighter—I'm talking about being one of the best, such as Anderson Silva. You have to look so good when you're fighting that people think you're not even trying. You have to look like you're capable of so much more, but if you were to pull it out, you'd start killing fools left and right. People are fascinated with this type of fighter. Though he's getting up there, Chuck Liddell had it for a while, but people forget fast.

But if you're not the supreme combatant with a crisp, smooth, and nearly unbelievable fight style that you can back up with the craftiness of a fox and catlike reflexes, don't fall into the trap of putting cosmetics before skills. Just be more like me, which is a guy who *seems* to work for everything. Show expression and how hard you're working in every movement. People get behind this type of fighter because you're acknowledging you're no better than they are— you're like a blue-collar guy just *trying* harder. You're a man of the people. You're Rocky. In *every* fight you want to be the underdog. Remind people in interviews before the fight that you're not a great athlete. You have to get them to invest emotions in you, which means being a likable, relatable-to person. Everywhere you go, you have to tell them that they have the prettiest women on the planet. You should also obey all their morals and local customs. For example, when in Alabama, you don't want to make jokes about the wrongness of sleeping with one's sister. They take offense at that.

Ways *Not* to Win the Crowd

1) Spit, urinate, or otherwise excrete upon them in any way. (Just trust me on this one.)

2) Make *any* sort of insulting remarks about their weather, women, or food. However, if you can include derogatory remarks about all three in the same sentence, you get a pass. For example, you can say, "I think this shitty weather and crappy food breeds ugly-ass women because I've seen a few monsters walking around this backwater town." If that backwater town happens to be a state capital, you get extra bonus points. This may not win the crowd, but you will win my heart, and maybe even a couple of seats at my next fight.

3) Fight a foreign fighter in his country. If you agree to scrap Georges St. Pierre in Montreal or Michael Bisping in England, label yourself the retarded villain.

4)   **Throw your jockstrap into the stands as though it's memora-
     bilia to fight over and cherish. If you do this and it *wins* crowd
     approval, cross that place off your "100 places to vacation" list.**

A Street Fight a Year
Could Get You a Beer

Street fighting—whether for a purse, turf, or pink slips (for you car douches)—is vastly different from fighting professionally in the ring or cage. For one, there are simply no rules on the street. Your opponent can kick you in the gonads, bite off your nose, try to tear off your ears, even defecate in his hand and throw a mud ball at you like a pissed-off howler monkey. If you try to fight like a gentleman and box by the Queensberry rules, there is a good chance your giblets will wind up in your throat. For this reason, my advice for street fighting is to tuck your head, put your hands up, and throw your fists as fast as you can from your chin to your opponent's chin as you move forward. You never want to back away—always move forward. When you've closed the distance and can't punch anymore, throw elbows. When you no longer have the room to throw elbows, deliver a series of head butts. This blind, fierce aggression is the best way to win a street fight, and I'm talking from experience . . . Oh shit, wait. I've lost a ton of street fights.

It's also important not to hesitate. Unless you're a social retard, you know when a fight is about to go down. I'm not talking about someone coming up to you and delivering a verbal beat-down, because people do this all the time and, often, it never comes to blows. I'm talking about when a punk's hands come up, his head drops, and he steps toward you with intent in his eyes. Instinctively, we all know what this means, but I don't know how many times I've seen the victim just stand there with his hands down and take the blow. It was like they were trying to convince themselves that somehow their instincts were wrong and they weren't just about to get punched in the face. In such a situation, you only have two choices—as the saying goes, fight or flight. If you decide to fight, do so hard and fast and without mercy. I've been in several scraps where I've tried to *half* fight my opponent, and it's plain stupid for two reasons: it gives your opponent an opportunity to land some good shots and it delays the conclusion of the scrap, which increases your chances of getting hauled off to jail. Once a fight starts, it starts. Go in fast and hard, cause your damage, and then get the hell out of Dodge.

If you're like most people and have an innate fear of fighting, the best way to get over it is to get into a couple of brawls. You don't want to go out and slap a guy who's eating dinner with his family because that's just fucked up, but you'd be surprised how easy it is to find a willing participant when in the mood to scrap. For example, I was sitting in a bar in Athens, Georgia, not long ago, and this kid comes up and gives me this funny look.

"Man, I would really like to fight you," he said.

"Yeah?"

"Yeah."

"Cool," I said. "Meet me in the bathroom in five minutes." It probably sounded gay (homosexual gay) to everyone else in the bar.

So after a couple of minutes, I head to the bathroom, and sure enough, he's in there waiting for me. I walk over to the sinks, take my watch off, put it in my hat, and then set my hat in the sink. I began shaking my arms out, waiting for this kid to back down and say something like, "Oh, I was just messing with you." After all, he wasn't a big dude, and he didn't appear to have much scrap in him. I kept waiting and waiting, and then I saw his hands go up and his feet move. *Shit*, I thought. *This kid has got some basic boxing. He seems to know what he's doing.* Without any hesitation, I rushed him. I hadn't realized that my friend Vern was at a urinal taking a leak. We crashed into him, causing him to piss everywhere. Not wanting to upset him any further, I pulled the kid into the clinch, he forced me against the wall, and I began dropping body shots as hard as I could with both fists. Eventually, I connected with a good one, he let a murmuring sound go, and then dropped into a heap on the floor. I went back to the sink, put my stuff back on, and then returned to the bar.

I told my friend Rory what had gone down, and he didn't believe me. "You're not some dumb-ass who gets into street fights in the bar bathroom," he said. "You're smarter than that."

"No, I'm not," I returned.

A few minutes later the kid comes up to me and outstretches a beer. "I saw you're drinking New Castle, and I bought you one."

"This is the kid I fought," I said to Rory.

"You just fight him?" Rory asked the kid.

"Yeah."

It was all so nonchalant. No one got seriously hurt, and no one had any hard feelings. The whole thing went so well that when a drunk college student asked me to wrestle in another bar later that night, I took him up on his offer. The funny part is that when I went back to Athens a year later and paid a visit to the Hardcore MMA gym, I saw both of these guys training. I'm pretty certain that they both had joined after our encounters, and I thought about asking the Hardcore Gym for some type of commission. Anyway, the moral of this story is that street fighting isn't that big of a deal, so there is no reason to let your fear hinder your going out to the bars with your old lady. If you get whomped on, so what. A black eye will disappear and a broken nose can be mended. Fear is a good thing because it keeps you alive, but if it becomes so great that it hinders you from doing what you want, you need to confront it head-on. . . . With that said, if you lose or get stabbed, I will tell everyone that I told you street fighting is stupid.

A Self-Defense Tip for the Ladies
(and the Prison Bound)

One of the best experiences of my life was when I taught a self-defense class to a group of freshmen law students at the University of Georgia. There were approximately thirty hot chicks in workout clothes, and I had them simulating raping one another. I kept shouting, "Come on, ladies, get your rape on!" But in all seriousness, it is important for women to learn at least some basic self-defense to protect themselves from the drooling perverts of the world. For the three women who've actually purchased this book, I've provided the "get up" move in the technique portion of this book that allows you to escape off your back. (If you are a dude who took my advice about getting into street fights to shatter your fear and are now being sent off to prison, you might also want to learn this technique to prevent, or at least *delay,* the inevitable man love you will receive in the other kind of cage.)

Dude, You Don't Always Have to Go Jackhammer

If you're passionate about fighting, you want to do everything in your power to prepare for a big bout. With your career and years of hard work on the line, it can be tempting to go to the gym three or four times a day. Although this can sometimes be beneficial, it is important to recognize when you are *overtraining*. If you don't listen to your body and continue to push yourself to the extreme, you'll do more harm than good.

Some of the Symptoms of Overtraining

1) **You've never felt this weak.**

2) **You're having trouble sleeping.**

3) **You experience a loss of appetite.**

4) **Weight loss beyond the norm.**

5) **Excessive muscle pain and cramping.**

6) **A noticeable loss in work capacity.**

7) **An abnormally high resting heart rate first thing in the morning. (In order to know that your heart rate is abnormally high, you must have a standard to judge by, which means monitoring your heart rate prior to your fatigued state.)**

8) **A curbed sex drive.**

If you've put a check mark next to all, most, or even *some* of the above, you're either admitting to overtraining or your best friends are Samuel Adams, Ben and Jerry, and your favorite watering hole is your couch (which is disgusting). But I don't know jack balls about Jenny Craig and how she helps fat people get their cottage-cheese thighs off the sofa, so let's go with "overtraining," which I know something about because I had this "friend" who found "himself" in this predicament . . .

Putting a stop to your training altogether is *not* the answer to restoring your virility, gentlemen. Instead, take a pause and try doing less of the most demanding exercises or drills in your regimen, replacing them with restoration training. For full-body fatigue or soreness, you'll want to do total-body activities, such as working out on the elliptical climber, an arc trainer, or a versa climber—something that involves both your arms and legs. The goal is to maintain a heart rate between a hundred and a hundred and twenty beats per minute for an extended amount of time to promote restorative blood flow throughout all peripheral links. Intensity is measured by your heart rate, so as long as you don't go above a hundred and twenty beats per minute, the intensity will place a very small demand on your body. If you get your heart rate too high, the energy demand changes. The next zone up from the restorative one is cardiac efficiency—go above that and you begin to work the aerobic system, and when your heart rate gets *really* high, it becomes anaerobic exercise. While it is important to routinely push your heart rate up to these levels, *you want to remain in the restorative zone until your fatigue dissipates.*

If you feel fatigued or overly sore in one particular muscle, you'll want to pick an exercise that replicates the particular movement that made you sore in the first place and perform excessive repetitions (this does not apply to beating off, for all you mad whackers). Just as with overall fatigue, you want to keep your heart rate between a hundred and a hundred and twenty beats per minute. When you do this exercise at a low intensity for an extended amount of time, you promote local blood flow to those specific tissues. For example, if your chest and arms are sore, you can get on the bench press and execute repetitions with just the weight of the bar. Of course how much weight you use is relative to how strong you are. At most, you want to do repetitions with 30 percent of the maximum weight you can press. The load should be heavy enough to stimulate the muscles, but light enough not to yield an excessive demand. When done properly, the local blood flow will restore your muscles and you'll be back to hard-core training in no time.

In addition to restoration exercises, it is also important to pamper your body when it's been overtrained. Personally, I follow the RICE recovery method, which is an acronym for rest, ice, compression, and elevation. Football trainers *live* by RICE. If you go to them with a broken ankle, all they'll say is, "Rice it, baby!" When my joints are sore, I'll frequently take ice baths because they cause the muscles to contract and squeeze out the lactic acid. Climbing into water that contains three twenty-pound bags of ice will undoubtedly shrink your cock 'n balls (or in my case, cock 'n ball—yes, I only have one nut) into a tightly constricted wad of cold turkey meat, but you always feel fresher coming out. I'll also do contrast baths, where I go back and forth between a cold tub of water and a hot shower.

Whether you've made the decision to become a professional fighter, an amateur fighter, or simply want to chisel your abs, which are now covered by a mound of cookie dough and lard, you have to take care of your body. It can be time-consuming and often inconvenient, but it's absolutely mandatory. For you pro-fighter wannabes, if you get into hand-to-hand combat with visions of fame and glory at the forefront of your half brain, you're in the wrong business, brother.

Training Is Like a Threesome—
(It's Best to Be in the Middle)

I like the idea of two chicks and one Forrest just as much as you do, Abner, Al, Billy Bob, and Butch. (Wondering how I knew your names? 'Cause if you're reading this, chances are your parents could only afford one page out of the baby-naming book, so the pickin's are slim.) But this section ain't about anything remotely sexual. And if that doesn't come across, chances are you screwed up the porn-mag section and the how-to book aisle again.

Training with the right group of guys is extremely important to becoming a successful mixed martial artist. You don't want to be the best guy in the room, nor do you want to be the worst. If you're the best, no one will push you, and you won't grow nearly as fast as you could. In some cases, you won't grow at all. On the flip side, you also don't want to be the worst guy in the gym because you'll only experience constant ass kickings. It's discouraging and your game will be built solely on defense. To get the most out of your training, you want to be the guy right in the middle. At Xtreme Couture, I'm that guy. I'll train with some of the less experienced guys to work positioning and my submissions, but then I'll roll with Robert Drysdale, a world-champion jujitsu practitioner, and work on my ability to survive against a superior grappler. I get my taste of victory, which keeps me motivated, and I also experience defeat, which pisses me off enough to push myself harder.

At some point, you may become the top dog in the gym, and it is important to be able to spot this changing of the guard. When it happens, you want to bring better people in to train with. This is what Randy Couture does—when training for a fight, he brings in people who are better than him in specific areas of fighting. If you don't have the luxury of doing this, the next best thing is to do rounds where you constantly rotate in fresh fighters. When you're gassed, a fresh fighter with half your skill has the ability to beat you, which in turn continues to promote growth. I know that becoming the best fighter in your camp is rewarding because it signifies all the hard work you've invested, but if you're a professional fighter, winning only counts in the cage. *Practice* is the time for learning and growing. It's time to push yourself beyond your limits and train your mind not to quit, and the only way you can accomplish this is to receive your fair share of beat-downs.

Filling the Holes . . . in Your *Game*, Spanky

Training the weakest part of your game requires the most willpower. For me, wrestling is undoubtedly the thing I suck at most when it comes to MMA. Unlike a lot of fighters, I haven't wrestled since I was two. My muscles aren't conditioned for the movements, and as a result I get dog-ass tired every time I do it. For the longest time, I ignored wrestling as though it were a nasty case of the crabs.

When the sport became my career, I quickly learned the importance of training the weakest part of your game, and I began forcing myself to wrestle on a regular basis. Over the past three years, I've noticed a sizable improvement. However, I probably would have made much larger gains had I not found escapes from this positive process of fixing holes in my game. The escape in question came in the form of injuries. If my elbow was acting up, the first thing I would skip was wrestling practice. You can bet your ass I suffered through striking and jujitsu practice, but when it came time to wrestle, my elbow would somehow suddenly hurt worse. *Fuck it*, I'd think, *I got to rest this injury. I'll pick wrestling back up when it gets better.*

The problem is that when you're a professional MMA fighter, you're injured all the time, and those injuries become an excuse to skip the parts of training you enjoy least. I'm not the only one who does it—I see it all the time with fighters. When Kale Yarbrough was on the *Ultimate Fighter* TV show, his knee was all jacked up. He is primarily a striker, and on the days we trained stand-up, he was right there in the mix, suffering through the pain. On the days we trained jujitsu, he'd sit out and nurse his injury.

If you don't have a fight coming up for four or five months, this is the wrong approach. The off-season should be spent on *improving* your weaknesses. Your time is actually very limited because a month or two before the battle, you should put your weaknesses aside and focus instead on fight-specific techniques. For example, if I have a fight coming up with a wrestler, two months before the bout I will spend my days perfecting the art of sprawling and escaping back to my feet should I get taken down. I'll spar with wrestlers and work on throwing punches as they come forward and kicks as they backpedal, but I won't spend nearly as much time actually wrestling because it's the last thing I want to do in the fight.

In order to continue to improve while injured, you've got to make sacrifices. If you're like me and wrestling is your primary weakness, go to wrestling practice but sit out when it's time to do striking. If you're a lousy kickboxer, go to striking practice and spar, but take a break when it comes time to wrestle. I have recently adopted this strategy, and although at times it's very difficult, I have noticed much larger gains in the areas of my game that need fixing.

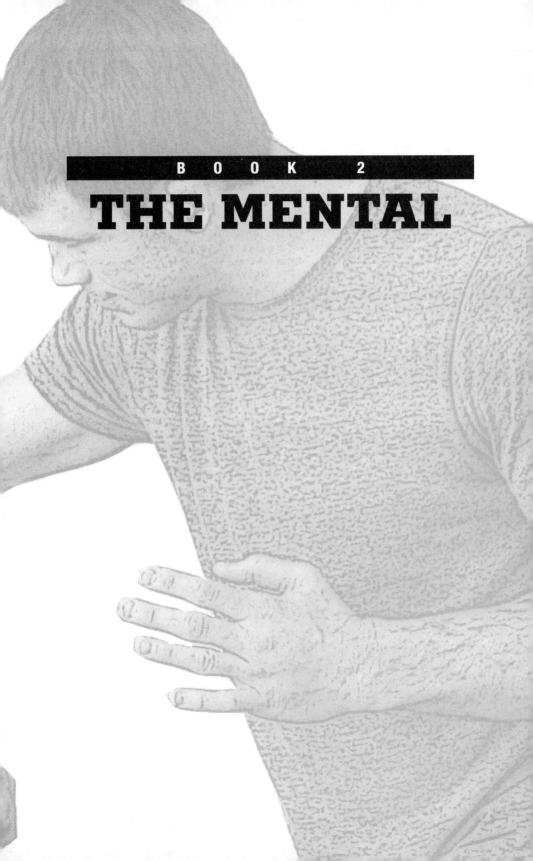

BOOK 2
THE MENTAL

We are dying from overthinking

—ANTHONY HOPKINS

He who hesitates, masturbates

—STOLEN BY FORREST FROM SOMEONE HE BEAT UP (HE'S PRETTY SURE)

If you overthink something long enough, you're almost guaranteed to suck at it big-time. For example, let's say the chick you've had a crush on since the second grade staggers up to you at a party and whispers in your ear, "I want you to screw my lights out." What do you do? You lead her to the nearest empty space and proceed to knock that ass out of the park. She experiences the best you can give, and you walk away feeling like a king. Now, let's say that same girl comes up to you on a Monday afternoon and says, "This weekend at the Christmas party, I want you to bang me stupid." If you're like most males, you smile, tap her confidently on one butt cheek, and immediately begin plotting all the nasty ways you will pleasure her. The problem is, nine times out of ten you don't come up with a solid game plan and then leave it, secure that your first effort is the right one. No, that would be far too simple. You play the scenario over and over again, perhaps even draw up a few diagrams. Come Friday afternoon, you've re-created the scene so many times that you're all fucked up in the head. You begin to doubt your ability to pleasure her at all. When it actually comes time to do the deed, performance anxiety has made you its bitch. That ass becomes a dark, alien world, and you stumble blindly through it searching for the G-spot. She goes away having experienced your absolute worst, and you go home feeling like a pissant, piece of shit, limp-dick motherfucker.

Overthinking a fight can be just as detrimental. When I was a kid, I won the first fight I ever got into because there was no time for analytical thought. The Billy badass of the school came up to me and socked me in the face, and I reacted by tackling him to the ground. I had no clue what the mount position was back then, but that's where I ended up. I delivered several stiff head butts to his face, busting him up and immediately causing him to break into tears. The teachers yanked me off him, but they didn't seem mad. They were too stunned. I was a quiet, nonviolent kid, yet I had just slapped a major beat-down on the school terror. Even the principal was shocked; all she could say was, "Don't do that again."

I didn't do that again, but it wasn't because I thought fighting was wrong. I was one of the only white kids in Monosana, an all-black school (I know, sooo cliché. If I ever meet Eminem, I'm going to punch him in the melon for ruining my "only white kid" bit), and if I had been a scrapping machine, I would have saved myself a lot of torment. The reason I didn't deliver any more ass kickings is that no one else stepped toward me with his fists clenched. They always approached me with trash talk, such as, "I'm gonna punch a hole through your face, bitch." Instead of analyzing if such an act was even possible, I would automatically believe him. I'd think, *Shit, this kid is gonna punch a hole in my face.* It didn't matter if he was half my size and the biggest wimp on the planet. I'd automatically back down. If that same kid had simply charged me, I probably would have turned his face into ground beef, but by talking shit, he gave me time to think about all the possible outcomes. I mean, come on, who wants to get a hole punched in their face? It was even worse when someone called me out early in the day, because then I'd sit there in class and think about it for the next four hours. By the time school got out, performance anxiety had turned me into the biggest bitch on the planet.

To prevent this from happening, never think about consequences before a fight. Throw rationality straight out the door. Of course, this is often harder than it sounds. By the time I made it to the UFC, I already had a number of fights under my belt, but that didn't stop me from overthinking my first few scraps. After all, I was in the UFC, hopefully fighting in front of millions of viewers. If I got my ass handed to me, I couldn't hunt down the five videotapes floating around, burn them, and be done with it. That shit would follow me around. I thought about every last detail and all the what-ifs a hundred times each and, as a result, I didn't perform to the best of my ability. A perfect example is my fight with Tito Ortiz—I overthought the hell out of that fight. Now, I'm not saying that you shouldn't game-plan for the fight. You need to do your homework, train as hard as you can every day, and know you won't quit on yourself. But as long as you cover those three bases, leave the coming fight behind you as you go about your business each day. A fight is just a fight, so don't make it any bigger in your mind. Remember, your life is small and meaningless.

Compartmentalization = Enlightenment
(Keeping Your Stools Solid)

A lot of people argue that mixed martial arts isn't a real job, and I would have to agree. If it were a real job, I wouldn't like it half as much. However, you can't say that because it's not a real job, fighters don't feel real stress. If you're just starting out in the sport, you're making at best five hundred dollars to step into the cage and five hundred dollars to win. It's possible to fight a couple of times a month, but only if you go uninjured. And if you always go uninjured, it probably means that you're quitting the instant the fight turns bad, making it damn near impossible to ever earn more than a thousand a fight. The money gets a little better if you make a name for yourself and get into one of the bigger shows, but then you've got autograph sessions and sponsorship photo shoots, and you have to travel all over the country to compete. You also have to contend with the stress of losing—tank two in a row, and you can find yourself back in the minor leagues.

An overload of stress can lead to an assortment of catastrophic side effects, the most disturbing ones being weight gain, poor immunity, decreased pain tolerance, constipation, rashes, gas, and massive testicular shrinkage. If you have a job that requires no human interaction, I suppose these side effects can be tolerable. But if you fight for money, the last thing you want is to be a fat, sick crybaby who is full of shit, always irritated, and passes gas into his training partners' faces while rolling. Throw a small package into the mix and you might as well shoot yourself in the face; repeatedly, if possible.

If you let these stresses get ahold of you, it ruins your training sessions, and if your training goes like crap, you'll most likely get your ass handed to you come fight night. In turn, the loss creates more stress, and soon you're on an Indian reservation in the bumfuck town of Clearlake, California, competing on the undercard of an IOU event. To shut down this negative stress cycle, I use a form of mental compartmentalization. For example, if it gets close to training time and I've got a long list of shit to do, I'll write it all down on a schedule and leave it sitting on the desk in my office, which happens to be my dining room table. By writing it down, I know it will be waiting for me when I get back, and can therefore clear my mind of everything on the list. If you keep that list in your head, not only do you risk forgetting shit, but you bring that list with you wherever you go, *including* the gym, and there goes your ability to focus on what you *need* to be doing.

I also apply compartmentalization techniques to the way I maintain my perspectives on fighting, training, and socializing. The instant I get to the gym, I leave the happy-go-lucky Forrest at the door and become a grade-A asswipe. If someone tries to talk to me about something other than the training ahead, I blow them off. It doesn't matter if it's a fan wanting an autograph or my dearest friend. If they push, I tell them very kindly, "Sorry, can't talk right now because I'm at work. I'd love to talk later." Personally, I don't feel this is rude. If I walked up to them while they were in the middle of their work, they'd probably tell me the same thing. It could be argued that because I'm a quasi-celebrity and depend on their patronage for my livelihood, the terms are different, and this point has a little merit. If someone approaches me on the street, I'll almost always stop to shoot the shit. Hell, I'll even take the time to strike up a conversation with someone if he or she approaches me while I'm in the middle of doing something most people consider important, like . . . say . . . purchasing my lady a wedding ring. If I'm not training, I'm the easiest guy in the world. I understand it can be jarring, making the transition from having the intense focus of a fighter to having a casual conversation, but I employ a technique called "verbal judo." My superiors taught it to me when I was on the police force in Georgia for when I'd be writing a report and some dipshit would come up and ask me a stupid question, like, "Is that gun real?" Verbal judo is basically a word that you say out loud or to yourself that allows you to quickly switch gears without blowing your lid. (It should be a peaceful word or sound, like *wooooosaaaaa*. You definitely don't want to make it an angry phrase, like "I'm going to stab you in the fucking eye!") So I'll do my best to be approachable on the street, but when I'm training, I try to turn the outside world off. If you're going to succeed in fighting, the gym has to be your inner sanctum, a place where you let your man out. And by "man out" I don't mean your penis. I mean the evil demon inside of you.

This form of compartmentalization also works the other way. When I step out of the gym for the day, I leave all thoughts of fighting behind me. Psychiatrists often say that you shouldn't do anything but fuck and sleep in your bed, and I wholeheartedly agree. I'm not one of those people who has UFC memorabilia plastered all over his house. I don't wear fight clothing outside of the gym, and I don't talk about fighting with my friends. Just as I make a list of all the bills I have to pay and leave it on my desk when I go train, I leave all the things I need to do to prepare for an upcoming fight on a schedule in the gym. This allows me to concentrate on what I'm doing, thereby reducing my stress. When I picture my home, I think of my cats, my old lady, good food, and watching movies. I don't even watch my opponents' fight tapes in the house—I do that between training sessions at the gym. My most prized hour each day is the one right before sleep. I'll just lie there with my woman, watching television and eating junk food. It doesn't matter if I had the crappiest training session of all time. In that hour, fighting doesn't exist.

Utilizing this form of compartmentalization doesn't mean you're denying your identity. If fighting is the primary focus of your life, it will obviously be a large part of who you are. It's the same as if you were a cop; you most likely hang out with other cops, tell cop stories, and go shooting once or twice a week. But just because you're a cop doesn't mean you have to wear the clothes every single cop on the planet wears when off duty. You don't need mug shots hanging up on your den walls or to watch only cop movies late at night. I truly believe that in order to excel in your profession, you need to have an identity outside of it. It's the only way to lessen the stress. A perfect example is my fight with Keith Jardine. I lost that bout, and as you could tell by my copious tears in the ring, I was pretty broken up (a moment of unmanliness, I'm sorry). But swear to God, when I walked out of the arena twenty minutes later, I was totally fine. I had a smile on my face and was bullshitting with my friends. If I didn't have an identity outside of the sport or lacked compartmentalization skills, I would have been devastated for a lot longer than the few moments I was holding my poor head after getting pounded upon, which in turn would have made it much more difficult to bounce back.

DICK IN A BOX

by Big John

Forrest doesn't just use visualization techniques to prepare for his fights—he also uses them to keep himself entertained. Back in 2000, he was working as a bouncer and struggling to complete a double major at the University of Georgia. Making just enough to hang on, he lived in a shitty, one-bedroom apartment. And when I say shitty, I mean shitty. The former tenant was a junkie or something, and left the place looking like a crack den. The landlord didn't want to clean up the mess, so he offered to waive Forrest's security deposit if he was willing to move in "as is." Forrest accepted, and it actually worked out in his favor because among the trash he found a brown leather jacket that he still wears to this day.

To personalize his hovel, Forrest brought in a 1970 television and accepted a mattress from Adam Singer. I know what you're thinking—how cool was that for Adam to help out a friend in need. No, it was not cool. The mattress was Adam's premarriage mattress from eight years prior, and since it had been spunked on more times than Courtney Love's hair, I'm seriously surprised it didn't sprout a pair of legs and walk away. The only other items Forrest had in the entire apartment (other than the former tenant's trash) were two pictures. One was of Martin Luther King Jr. and the other was of Clint Eastwood—his two idols.

After a workout one afternoon, Forrest and me headed over to his place for a protein shake. We're sitting there on the floor, staring at the 1970 television, and he proceeds to tell me that he sometimes gets lonely and has conversations with me when I'm not there. I thought he was joking, but then he proceeds to tell me all about some of the great conversations that we'd had. He didn't go so far as to say, "remember the time . . ." or "that was hilarious when you said . . ." but he went on and on about how clever some of the things my imaginary self had said. At that point, most normal people would have looked carefully around the apartment, noticed the 1970 television, the stained mattress on the floor, and the two pictures on the walls, and realized that in fact they were sitting in the apartment of a serial killer in the making, but I'm a few parts crazy myself. All I could do was smile. I had always realized Forrest was nuts—I had just never realized how nuts. When he failed the psychological test for the Gainesville Police Department about a year later, I wasn't surprised in the least.

FORREST'S REPLY

It's quite comical that Big John thinks I'm insane because he's the craziest fucker on the face of the planet. I can prove this with a few simple stories. A few days after the Virginia Tech massacre in 2007, he was lying naked in bed at two in the morning, drunk as shit, watching a Renzo Gracie instructional video. You might think it strange that he was viewing a training video naked, but John refuses to wear clothes inside, ever . . . Starting to get the picture? So anyway, his apartment building catches on fire, causing the sprinklers to go on. As a federal police officer and a gun lover, he has all sorts of expensive weapons lying around his abode. Not wanting them to take water damage, he squeezed his 290-pound naked body into a pair of jeans, strapped his AR-15 over one shoulder, his shotgun over the other shoulder, and tucked his two Glocks into his pants, which he was unable to button because of his massive belly. Next, he put on his Georgia Tech football ring and his two ATT Championship rings. Did I mention his toenails were painted black? Yeah; well, they were. Instead of taking the time to put on a shirt and a pair of shoes, he grabbed a twelve-pack of beer from the refrigerator. Feeling he had covered all the bases, he headed out onto his balcony and went barreling down the fire escape.

As John was going down, a group of firemen were walking up to the scene. This is the image they saw: a 290-pound man armed with an assault rifle, a shotgun, and two handguns, sliding down a fire escape with no shirt, no shoes, black toenails, carrying a twelve-pack of beer. When John reached the bottom of the fire escape, instead of identifying himself as an officer of the law, he gave the approaching fireman a drunken smile. Remember, this is just two days after a gunman went ballistic at Georgia Tech, killing thirty-two people. Immediately all the firemen assumed he had started the fire and had been waiting for them to show up to kill them. One fireman shit himself. And I don't mean figuratively—I mean he literally shit himself.

Failing to pick up on the fact that he was scaring the shit out of people, John walked over to the curb, laid his guns out next to him, and then cracked a beer. A few minutes later, cops swarmed around him with their guns drawn, ordering him down on the ground. After a few seconds, one of them recognized him.

"John, is that you?" the cop shouted.

Visualize
(or, What the Hippie Chicks Taught Me)

The closer you get to a fight, the more it will weigh on your mind. If a few days before a show I find myself unable to leave thoughts of the fight at the gym, I'll use a visualization technique to clear my mind. It's pretty simple, which is fitting since I learned it at basketball camp when I was thirteen. All you do is draw a bath, climb inside, and then go over all the possible outcomes, both good and bad. Once you've run through every possible scenario, pull the plug and visualize all your worry and anxiety running down the drain with the water. After all the water goes out, hop in the shower and clear your head of all thoughts of the fight. I've done this on several occasions, and it works surprisingly well.

A similar technique can also be used to switch your brain from "fucking-around mode" to "training mode" before practice. About twenty minutes before I head to the gym, I'll jump in the shower. The instant the water hits me, I think of all the little things I need to accomplish that day and the little victories I need to have. After the shower, I drink an Americana espresso from Starbucks (please, please sponsor me!). When the coffee is finished, it signifies that it's time to work. (If Starbucks does not sponsor me, screw drinking coffee as a part

"Yeah, it's me, it's me, it's me."

If that story isn't enough to convince you that he doesn't have his head screwed on quite right, let me tell you about the movie character he most likes to impersonate. It's not Al Pacino or Dustin Hoffman—it's Buffalo Bill from *The Silence of the Lambs*. The first time I brought my wife over to his place to meet him, he answered the door doing this impersonation. Butt-ass naked with his junk tucked between his legs, he began a slow dance and said, "Would you fuck me? . . . I'd fuck me." And this is how sick he is—he replayed that part of the movie over and over, practicing the dance until he had it just right. Yeah, and I'm the disturbed one.

of your routine. Drink a protein shake instead.) The little routine is what I've heard physiologists call a Phase Changing Activity, which is something that allows you to make a transition from one mind-set to another. (Yeah, my IQ is above 67, asshole . . . It's 87. No fucking kidding, that's the IQ score I got in college. Is that good?) It doesn't have to be a shower and a coffee—it could just as well be a shit and a screw, and not necessarily in that order. I find it extremely helpful because going from the tranquillity of your home to the adrenaline-charged gym can at times be very jarring. The smoother the transition, the better training will go.

If It Looks Like a Poser, and Smells Like a Poser . . .

A while ago, a *New York Times* reporter wrote an article about a new trend sweeping the nation—teenage boys bending and pulling on their ears with the intention of snapping the cartilage and developing the nasty, pus-filled lumps often referred to as cauliflower ear. According to the reporter, their goal is to appear cool, like professional mixed martial artists. Personally, I don't think this is a trend. I think the reporter visited one gym, and that gym was located in some bumfuck town in the Appalachian Mountains. He approached an inbred kid sitting on the street out front, and the conversation went something like this:

"Hello, my name is Dipshit and I'm a reporter from the *New York Times*. I'm doing a story on the new sensational sport of mixed martial arts, and I would like to interview you."

"Uh, art is for faggots," the kid said. "Mama says so."

"That's great. So how many times a week do you roll?"

"I used to roll every day, but then Mama ate all my Ecstasy. Rollin' is cool."

"Great," the reporter said, scratching in his pad. "We'll say five times a week. Now, I noticed that your left ear is mangled. You have what they call cauliflower ear in the industry. Was that self-inflicted to appear cool? You know, like all the big grown-up fighters that you look up to? Guys like Randy Couture?"

"In . . . Inflic . . . What you say?"

"Did you do that to yourself? Your ear."

"Oh, hell yeah. Sure did. I was rollin' pretty good, and then I blacked out and my face fell into the hotness of the stove. The glowing part."

"Great. So you train at home as well. Real dedication. Do all your friends do that to their ears?"

"Most. Those of us who roll, we tend to fall into a lot of things that are hot. Sometimes our papas help us with it. You know, hold our faces down into those square things that make water bubble."

"So your parents encourage you with this ritual. Interesting. Would you call it a trend that is sweeping the nation?"

"I ain't sweepin' shit! Get outta here now, ya hear!"

"Never mind. I got my story. Thanks, kid."

I seriously hope that this is the way it went down. If the reporter actually did his homework (which I highly doubt, considering the journalistic integrity of Philip Glass), and busting up your ears has truly become a trend sweeping the male youth of America, there are a lot more fake-ass, Poindexter douche bags out there than I thought. First off, you don't need cauliflower ear to be a fighter. Kale Sanders, a world-championship wrestler, doesn't have cauliflower ear, and he's one of the biggest badasses on the planet.

**If You're a Little Pussy but Want to *Appear* Tough,
You Don't Have to Go So Far as Busting Up Your Ears.
You Only Need to Accomplish Six Things**

1) Get some letters shaved into your hair, all the way down to the scalp, and then have your stylist, Roy, finish off your do with a fabulous multicolor dye job! (Happy Ending optional☺ [fighters love emoticons].)

2) Acquire a number of those really cool tattoos that everyone has: barbed-wire armbands (you know, the ones that chicks got in 1995?), a really scary skull, or simply have your name (or the nickname that your gang gave you when you jumped in on the supermean streets of Malibu) inked on with that really hard-looking calligraphy-type stencil stuff. The grenade on the side of the neck is always good, but putting one on your biceps is just as good as long as you wear a Tap Out tank top. FYI, biceps tattoos look really cool when your gunboats are all swollen from blasting out curls.

3) Some sort of fight-related T-shirt. If you don't have one, then you need a T-shirt that has something to do with guns—HK, PRO-TECTED BY GLOCK, something that will most definitely strike fear into the hearts of men at a glance. As an added bonus, you might want to throw in some leather wristbands, or at least something wristband-looking, like a watch with a really wide strap—a Swatch on a wristband! There ya go.

4) A number of noticeable body piercings. (If they are unnotice-able, like a Prince Albert, then you are gross.) Although the majority of real fighters don't have piercings because they get ripped out during training, the fans don't take the time to think of this occupational hazard, allowing you (the would-be con-tender) to sport these tantalizing, first-strike targets to any of us who might actually engage you in a brawl.

5) Make sure you write the word *fighter* as your occupation on ALL legal documents. This includes lease agreements, health plans, or the application for your brand-new job at Jiffy Lube. Word to the wise: only NON-posers write self-employed.

6)   This book, *Got Fight?* (available now online and in your favorite local bookstore, including, but not limited to: Amazon.com, Borders, Barnes & Noble, Fred's Deli, Xandi's fish market on the corner of Thirty-third and Twelfth near the old rusted Dumpster, you know the one . . . where Sheila works? Ahhh . . . Magic Lips Sheila . . . Anyway . . .), must be in your hands at all times, and when in public, you want to open it up and pretend to read. This will cause hot, really dumb chicks to come up to you and ask if you fight, because these fine specimens are overly dumb and will sleep with you. If you can indeed throw down, you should clap my book shut, throw it aside, and say, "That guy don't have nothing to offer about fighting I don't already know. Wanna see my grenade tattoo?"

7)   Finally, and perhaps the most dangerous of all, make sure to pronounce the word *jujitsu* in your fanciest Portuguese accent. (Sarcasm aside, because you bought this book, I like you and will maintain that position until you do some stupid homoerotic prank shit like they do on *The Ultimate Fighter,* so a serious word to the wise—and the stupid: when in the presence of a true Brazilian, do NOT try to pronounce this sacred word in such a fashion, as you will receive an expeditious ass-whoopin' that you had not previously thought physically possible—I present Mr. Wanderlei Silva, the Axe Murderer—get it, Fuck Face?)

8)   Even if you say you're going to list six things, like I did above, always list more. The fact that you've lost your ability to count is verification enough that you are a fighter. And if your list mixes numbers and letters in the way it's organized—as in *item 1, item b*—most people will think you once held a championship belt of *some* sort.

If you are indeed capable of accomplishing all eight of the requirements on the above checklist, I guarantee with absolute certainty that you will realize the look and notoriety of a professional, Richard Grieco–class douche bag. At such point, your value as a human being will solely depend upon your ability to actually convince people you are a true badass. Back in the day, this could only be done by the big guys, but no longer. Thanks to the weight divisions added a few years ago, it doesn't matter how small you actually are. Hurray! If you weigh a buck ten, just tell people you compete in the WEC.

As you now know, there is no reason to mangle your ears. The only reason you'd want to do this is if you fear another fight poser fucking with you in a bar. In such a case, the fatter your ears, the less likely he will be to punch or kick you. My point is, why stop there? If your goal is to intimidate, you might as well develop cauliflower face. I doubt you've ever seen me up close, and that is a good thing. I have an extra bump on my nose, scar tissue above and below both eyes, tic-tac-toe marks all across my face, and two massive cauliflower ears that protrude off the side of my head. When you get up into my grille, there is only one thing that crosses your mind: *Man, this goofy bastard has got the shit beat out of him before. And here he is walking around with a smile on his face like he owns the joint. Maybe I shouldn't mess with him.*

Developing cauliflower face, like me, is a lot harder than developing cauliflower ears. If you're unwilling to actually receive these facial scars and markings through training, it requires you to repeatedly run that stupid face straight into the corners of various walls and doorways. So I would suggest just checking off the eight things above and leaving it at that. Just don't forget to carry around my book—that part is superimportant. As a matter of fact, tell all your friends to also pick up a copy. By now, it's probably on the five-dollar rack, and what's five bucks?

Treating That Ear

If you end up getting cauliflower ear through legitimate means that can be verified by the guy or guys who did it to you (i.e., through training) and don't give a shit about looking like an ugly-ass professional fighter, you will want to drain those kumquats before they get too big. If you don't have an idea of what too big is, take a look at the Cage Rage fight between James Thompson and Kimbo Slice. Thompson's ears were so large it looked like shaved bulldog balls were stuck to the sides of his sweaty head (and when they exploded midfight, they looked like—no, no, it's too painful to say, and brings back many bad memories). There are a couple of ways to drain cauliflower ears. The safest method is to go to the doctor, but this doesn't always work out. One time (God,

I feel like I'm confessing STDs or something), I went to the doc to get my ears drained and he was a major fuckhead.

"Are you going to quit wrestling for a month if I do this?" he asked.

"No, of course not."

"Then you might as well go."

Thanks a lot, asswipe.

The second method is the good ol' DIY, which requires a few supplies: a bottle of rubbing alcohol, a bottle of drinking alcohol, Neosporin, and a syringe—a *clean* syringe (i.e., not used by junkies). Back in the long-time-ago time, my training partners and me all used the same syringe. We'd burn the tip with a lighter, dunk it in some rubbing alcohol, and call it safe. Seriously. We'd seen junkies do it in the movies, so we figured it had to work. Sometimes I *am* as stupid as I look.

Anyway, if you don't have a *clean* syringe, you'll want to use some type of knife—hopefully not one you've recently used to clean fish, but one you'd imagine being perfect for draining, say . . . bulldog balls.

Once you have all the supplies, put the rubbing alcohol on your ear, poke a small hole in your cauliflower, and then squeeze the pus out with your fingers. You won't want to cover it up afterward, because over the next several hours you will continue to experience leakage. However, it is essential to smear on a heap of Neosporin to prevent infection caused by the syringe (which, despite my warning, was probably used by a heroin addict or two) or the bulldog-ball-splitting blade.

The Smack Attack

When you get into a confrontation on the street, talking trash can be a very valuable tool. This is especially true when you know your aggressor will most likely smash your face in, should you come to blows. The crazier you sound, the less likely he will be to throw a punch. Below, I've included a few examples of how to verbally strike your opponent for intimidation purposes.

1) **"Be careful, son, I'm bathed in the devil's menstrual blood!"**
    (An oldie, but goodie.)

2) "You creeping up on the 963, sucka?" (This has a very gang-sterish feel and, for this reason, should not be used when your aggressor is a gangster. If you do, you will probably get shot. The numbers are not important—but there should always be three to represent an area code. However, you do not want to use the area code that applies to your current location or the thug staring you down will know you are full of shit and proceed to pummel your face.)

3) "I lick a dog's ass with guys like you." (This has many levels of intimidation. First, it's confusing, and anything that is confusing tends to be a little scary. Second, it involves a dog's ass. It will lead your attacker to wonder if you like dogs' asses, and if you do, are you going to rape him after you beat him. It's more than a sane mind can handle.)

4) "Naw, naw, naw. You don't get to fight me. You got to fight my bitches first. If you can get through them, you get a piece of me." (This makes you sound really cool. If you have more than one chick, you're a pimp or a player. Either way, no one will want to beat you up. They will want to make you their friend.)

5) "I fuck guys like you in jail." (It helps to drool while screaming this.)

It is important to learn these types of verbal attacks to avoid confrontations on the street, but when it comes to professional fighting, talking trash serves very little purpose. It doesn't matter if you call your opponent the son of a crack whore or praise the ground he walks on—come fight night, he is going to try to knock your head off your shoulders and break your arm just the same. If anything, trash talk will only motivate your opponent during training. Repeating your words over and over in his mind, he might find the juice to stay in the gym an hour longer than he otherwise would have. Remembering the nasty shit you said about his hygiene or his mother might encourage him to spend more time reviewing your tapes. I could see doing it if you got something on your end, but you don't. Unless you've received trash-talk training from professional wrestlers in the WWE, the majority of the time you come off sounding mildly retarded. With that said, I have to admit that I've seen a calm, cool, matter-of-fact form of trash talk work on one occasion, but it really was more of a sign of utter confidence than a form of shit talking. It was at the press conference before Chuck Liddell took on Babalu Sobral. There were more than a hundred people there, all staring up at these two fighters.

"How do you see this fight going?" a reporter asked Liddell.

Liddell looked out over the crowd, and without a trace of emotion or an ounce of cockiness in his voice, he said, "I'm going to knock Babalu out."

The way he said it made it sound as if it had already happened or he had somehow looked into the future and seen the outcome. Half the crowd immediately began nodding their heads, confirming the knockout. The other half glanced over to Babalu, and judging by the look on his face, he, too, was convinced. Although he didn't come right out and say it, you could almost hear him thinking, *Yeah, he's probably going to knock me out.* It was psychological warfare at its finest. It probably wouldn't have worked so well if Chuck had never won a fight, but at the time he was KING at knocking people out. If it's your first fight, don't talk trash. It will only make you look like a jackass if you should get beaten in the first four seconds. It will also inspire your opponent to cackle as he does a victory dance around your fallen body. Not good for your highlight reel.

Things Not to Say Before a Professional Fight

1) I'm going to kick his ass.

2) I'm going to beat his head in.

3) I'm gonna mess his face up so his mama don't recognize him.

4) I'm gonna whoop him so severely his girlfriend's ovaries fall out.

5) I'm going to man up!

You get the point—basically any of the ass-kicking clichés. If you need more examples of what not to say, just watch a WEC fight. Those guys are absolute masters at how to trash talk poorly.

If the Interviewer Is Forcing You to Say Something,
Instead of Talking Trash, Use a Generic Sports analogy

1) I'm going to give a hundred and ten percent. I don't know how that's humanly possible, but I'll find a way.

2) I'm going to do my best, give it all I got.

3) I won't quit until the bell.

4) He's going to know he's in a fight.

Let Me See That Big-Nut Strut

Mixed martial arts is a difficult sport to judge due to its complexity. For each round, the judges must observe and absorb a huge amount of information, including strikes, takedowns, submission attempts, and Octagon control, which, in total, is a fancy way to say *aggression*. If it's an extremely close fight, at the end of a round an inexperienced judge (of which there are many) will likely be unable to compute all the data, causing him to refer to the fighters' appearance and general attitude when filling out the scorecard. As a result, you must pay special attention to how you *behave* after each round.

Personally, I use the system created by the renowned Cleveland Brown's running back Jim Brown. When he played football, he got up slow after every play, casually handed the ball to the referee, and then walked gingerly back to the huddle. It didn't matter if it was the first quarter or the fourth—he had the same expression on his face and walked at the exact same speed. His coach eventually asked him why he didn't pop up and put a hustle in his stride, and Jim's answer was simple.

"Then what happens after I've carried the ball thirty times and can no longer hustle back? I'll tell you what—the other team sees that I'm walking, that I'm weak, totally done. I'd be giving away my ace right there." (My editor asked me if these were the exact words that Jim Brown used, and my answer was, "Haven't a fucking clue." I was just trying to tell a story, you know? I think I remember him saying something kind of like that, but things tend to get a little funny in my head. Thanks, Adam Korn, for completely breaking up this little tale. Way to go, buddy.)

It's quite genius if you think about it. By hiding his energy and enthusiasm when he had it, he could make people think he had energy and enthusiasm when he didn't. People watching him for the first time might look at his sluggish movements and think him either lazy or exhausted, but after seeing him climb back to his feet in a calm and collected manner a dozen times, they get used to his speed. It begins to appear normal.

Although Jim Brown devised this tactic for the game of football, it works just as well in mixed martial arts. It can be used to mask your weakness from your opponent, your opponent's cornermen, the fans in the crowd, and, most importantly, the judges who are scoring your bout. If a fight ends and I'm in a dominant position, I'll casually disengage and walk nice and easy back to my corner. This is often difficult to accomplish after the first round because my adrenaline is through the roof, but I'll force myself to slow down in order to set a standard in the minds of those watching. The only way I'll increase my speed is if a round ends and I'm stuck in a bad position. In such a case, I will pop up quickly to show the judges that I'm physically all right, and then walk casually back to my corner. By the end of the fifth round, when walking is all I can manage, I appear just as fresh as when the fight started.

While it can certainly make a positive impression in the minds of the judges if you rush back to your corner and choose to stand rather than sit, fights are generally determined by how they end rather than how they start, so you better rush back to your corner and stand after every single round. If you no longer have the energy to do both, it tells the judges that you have been broken. It doesn't matter if your opponent is also too weak to stand—if he's been walking back to his corner and sitting between every round, there is no way to determine if he is tired or not. So take my advice and relax the instant the bell sounds. Even though no points are being scored during the intermissions, you're being judged. *Consistency* is the way to prevent that judgment from working against you.

Consolidation Prevents Constipation

When I went out with a group of guys from the Hardcore Gym in Athens, Georgia a few years back, I made a bet that I could eat a hundred Buffalo wings at a local dive bar. Now, I've always thought training for fights was rather easy, so I figured the eating challenge would also be easy. And, for the most part, it was. I consumed fifty wings down to the bone, and felt Massengill fresh! We had all sorts of cool stuff planned that night, but I figured I would polish off the remaining fifty before we headed out. However, the batch of twenty-five wings the waitress put before me were spicy. I don't do well with spicy things, and my friends knew this. To help me wash down the fiery meat, they began feeding me pitchers of New Castle, which is one of the thicker beers. After I had downed two pitchers, they began purchasing me chocolate martinis, thinking the sugar would wake me up. I had three of them. By the time I made it to seventy-five wings, I *no longer* felt Massengill fresh. With pounds of meat swimming in a soup of beer and chocolate martinis, there was no way I could consume the rest or even head out for our debaucherous night on the town. I was so sick, I had to lie down on the floor of the bar for several hours. I kept mumbling over and over, "Oh God, I made a mistake," and vociferously promised sweet baby Jesus I would never ever accept an eating challenge again.

But, in hindsight, the mistake I made wasn't in *accepting* the challenge; it was in taking advice from my jerkwad friends. If I had had my senses about me, I would have realized that drinking a river of heavy beer and hard alcohol would hinder my primary objective, but when you're in the thick of battle, rationality rarely steps into the picture. When you're tired and slightly worn down, outside advice always seems like good advice. After all, it's a different perspective, and your mind somehow convinces you that this other perspective is clearer and better than yours.

This type of derailment doesn't just happen in the realm of childish bets— it happens all the time in fighting. You've got grappling coaches, striking coaches, strength and conditioning coaches—you've got all these coaches who have opinions on what you should and should not be doing. Having so many coaches in your arsenal helps when you're a member of a well-organized gym because the trainers tend to work together to develop your regimen, but, on occasion, things can turn into an egofest. Each trainer knows his individual field better than the others, and his natural inclination is to steer you toward becoming a master in his arena. But the more you work on one aspect of fighting, the less you can work on the others. If all of your coaches are like this, you'll quickly become overtrained. To prevent this from happening, it is important to *constantly* monitor your workouts. If you feel you are being pushed too hard in one aspect, instead of going along with it, you need to get your coaches together to have a meeting. This can often be a difficult thing to ask for because you view yourself as the student and your trainers as your teachers, but if they are good coaches, they will have your best interest at heart. These meetings can get rather intense, even produce a long-winded argument as to what's more important, so I strongly suggest sitting them out. Let them figure things out among themselves, and be open to hearing what they *collectively* suggest. If they can't agree on a unified regimen and your training suffers, you know they're only out for themselves and you're training at the wrong gym.

You Know How to Judge the Size of a Man's Genitals? By Looking at Defeat
(Note: Never be concerned about another man's genitals unless he used to fuck your old lady)

It doesn't matter if you have the slickest submissions on the planet and possess the strength of a silverback gorilla—if you compete for long enough in mixed martial arts, you're going to get beat. When this day comes, it is important to take a hard look at yourself and your training. If you did everything in your power to train for the fight and just got knocked the fuck out, don't sweat it. It happens to the best of the best. After a loss, it's natural to experience a sick feeling in the pit of your stomach and find it difficult to look into people's eyes, but if that feeling persists, it's usually because your mind is trying to tell you something. You need to ask yourself, *Did I take it serious enough? Did I eat all the right things? Did I train all aspects of fighting hard enough?*

To discover what you can do better the next time around, review the fight tape and analyze your performance. It can suck to watch yourself get put to sleep by a hard right over and over, but it is the only way to know if those voices whispering in the back of your head have any merit. I watched my fight with Jardine, and I didn't like what I saw. Every time I broke away from the clinch, I'd step toward my right, directly into the power of his left hand. To make matters worse, I'd do so with my hands down, giving him a free shot at my face. The other thing I didn't like was the form of my kicks. Going into the fight, I knew he would throw a lot of leg kicks, and I was determined to outkick him and break him down in that area of the fight. The problem was that every time I threw a kick, I would again drop my hands. The combination of these mistakes allowed Jardine to land that one big blow and put me down. That sleeping pill was a stern wake-up call. When training for a fight, it's easy to convince yourself that you're training all the right things and as hard as you possibly can, but after a loss, the proof is always right there on the screen. And it's not about how hard you try, but about what some call *deliberate* practice—the practice that improves your game and makes you great.

I went back to the drawing board and focused on all the little details that I had previously missed or cast aside. If you watch my next fight, which was against Hector Ramirez, anyone could see just how much of a difference these small improvements made. I broke down every aspect of my training, and the result was clean, crisp combinations that landed a large percentage of the time. Of course, everything is a learning process, and you can't expect to get it all right your first time around. If you try something and it doesn't work, instead of getting discouraged, go back to the drawing board.

You'll often hear fighters say that losing was the best thing that could have happened to them, and if you're a guy who uses defeats to get your shit together, most of the time it's the truth. UFC fighter Martin Kampman is a perfect example. When he first came to Xtreme Couture, I'd submit him like it was nothing. Instead of getting discouraged, he'd analyze what he did wrong, and then go off and grapple with someone who was even better than me. At first, I thought he was some type of masochist. But then I began to notice massive improvements in his game, and in a very short period of time. By viewing his losses as victories, he pinpointed his weaknesses, and then he did everything in his power to eradicate those weaknesses. As a result, he improved faster than anyone else in the gym. Adopting this kind of mind-set will drastically improve your game. If you choose a hardheaded, know-it-all mind-set instead, chances are you'll always make the same mistakes—and you'd better hope that you never fight me because if I watch your tapes and notice you overtly making the same mistakes you made in prior fights, I will exploit you like a motherfucker. But you can thank me when we're lying next to each other in the hospital because I'll have given you a free lesson in up-ping your game.

Be Humble, Grasshopper

I'm not sure if I'm humble, have a really good self-understanding, or just have a tremendous amount of self-loathing. All I know is that I can see what I am as well as what I am not. I realize I've had some good fights, but I have never fought miraculously like Anderson Silva or BJ Penn. I've never had a reign of terror like Chuck Liddell. And the reason is simple—I'm not as gifted as those guys. I push my body and mind to their limits in training, but I'm not so delu-sional that I think I'm the best fighter to have ever walked the planet.

Being honest with yourself is the best way to live life because it keeps you from having massive falls. After all, if you think you are unbeatable, and then get your ass served to you on a platter, your whole world comes crumbling down. That's when the excuses start to flow, but who is buying them? No one. Not yourself, not others. If you can admit to yourself that you simply got beat by a better fighter, it dissolves the lies and allows you to be a happier person.

Although it can be depressing to admit to yourself that you will never be the best, it is liberating at the same time. Instead of trying to be better than everyone else, which is existentially arrogant, you can focus on being the best that *you* can be. Even if you can never defeat the Anderson Silvas and BJ Penns of the world, you can take pride in the fact that you did the most you possibly could with what you were given. You can take pride in every accomplishment. What more can you ask for? Wishing that you were three inches taller or that your dick would grow an extra five inches delivers nothing but misery, brother.

If you choose to ignore this advice and treat the world as though you own it, when you do fall, everyone is going to kick you while you're down. If you're *humble* in defeat, everyone may still kick you, but they won't kick you as much.

Blooooooood

There are a lot of hemophobiacs running around out there. And no, I'm not re-ferring to people who have a fear of man-on-man love. A hemophobiac is someone who can't handle the sight of blood. There are varying degrees of this phobia. Some people simply get an uneasy feeling at the sight of blood, while others actually experience a decrease in heart rate and blood pressure, causing them to pass the fuck out. If you think about all the thousands of different phobias circling around, it makes more sense than most. People who *have* this condition fear blood because it reminds them of their vulnerability and mortality, and that doesn't seem to be a bad thing to be concerned about. Certainly makes more sense than getting freaked out by two guys who enjoy playing ass darts in the privacy of their own home.

Personally, I've never had issues with blood. A part of it probably has to do with the fact that I got my ass kicked on a regular basis as a kid. And when I say "regular basis," I mean every week. Seriously, I got my ass kicked so many times in Georgia's public school system, my mother ended up sending me to Catholic school. (Sorry about all the cursing in this book, Sister Margaret.) There is, however, an upside. After the local bullies turn your face into a piñata half a dozen times, you begin to realize that spilling a little blood doesn't mean you're teetering on the verge of life and death. Even when you leave a good-size puddle of your life fluid (the *other* life fluid, moron) on the pavement, you understand that you're still nowhere close to taking the Long Sleep Good Night.

By the time I made it to high school, getting beat up and bleeding was just a part of the routine. One of my bloodiest ass-whoopings occurred in the locker room before basketball practice. I was suiting up with the team, and the super-stud jock that had made it his life purpose to fuck with me began going on and on about how my shirt was too tight and my shorts were too short. He had been riding me for years, and something snapped. I knew his mother had recently died, and so I turned to him and said the most fucked-up thing I could possibly say.

"Does that make you feel better?" I asked, looking at him in the eyes. "Does it take your mind off the fact that the maggots are eating your mother right now?"

Pretty fucked up, I know. But I was tired of being punked. He instantly tackled me down and started beating the holy hell out of me. I was stuck between a bench and the lockers, and I didn't even *try* to defend myself. As he hit me over and over in the face, I just laughed my ass off because I knew that no matter how hard he hit me, I had gotten the better of him. No amount of physical pain could equal what I had just done to him. The other players in the locker room didn't know what the hell was going on, so they pulled him off of me. My nose was jacked up pretty bad and blood was everywhere, but it obviously wasn't that big of a deal because I couldn't stop laughing.

It's probably best not to attempt to acquire my whimsidaisical attitude toward blood because it will most likely lead to a lack of concern for getting your ass kicked, which in turn can lead to a fucked-up face like mine. But if you plan on fighting, a fear of blood is sort of a setback. Err on the side of loving it like Penn. I've seen a lot of fighters who have that fear—the instant they receive a small cut, they begin dabbing at their face and checking their hand. Sometimes their knees grow weak, and other times they simply give up. Seriously, I've seen guys give up from a small cut, and I'm not just talking about in the old days. I've also seen fighters overreact when they open up a cut on their opponent. Instead of seeing the cut for what it was—a small laceration in their opponent's skin that does absolutely nothing to hinder his ability to fight (unless, of course, it's above the eyes)—they behave as though the opponent is hanging on to life by a thread, and go crazy with strikes, leaving themselves exposed to counterattacks. (Personally, I would much rather bleed than my opponent because I don't know where he's been. I've seen the kind of women some of the fighters fuck, and it's scary.)

The bottom line is that neither you nor your opponent is going to bleed out in the ring. The average adult male has approximately ten pints of blood in his body. Lose one pint, and you might feel a little light-headed. Lose two pints, and you'll probably feel a little dizzy and perhaps a slight chill. It's not until you lose three pints that your body begins to shut down. How much is three pints? Well, it's three pints. But that's a fucking lot of blood. The chance that you'll bleed even a pint out of a cut on your head is pretty damn rare, so if you start to feel queasy or think that your heart is beginning to fade, it's just in your mind. Trust me, the referee will stop the bout long before you bleed to death. If not, then at least you'll be the first.

Now, if you receive a cut, you want to tend to it afterward as quickly as possible. You might *think* it would look cool to have a lump of scar tissue above one eye, but scar tissue is weaker than skin, and chances are it will open up again the next time you get punched. Take my face, for example—I've got scars all over the damn thing, and all you need to do is touch my face for it to start bleeding, which leads those watching my fights to think that my opponent has superhuman power in his punches, when in fact my face will open up under the pressure of a decent-size yawn. To keep from becoming a "bleeder," you want to get your cuts stitched up. If you're competing in the UFC or one of the other larger promotions, they will most likely take proper care of you. However, it's not this way in a lot of the smaller shows. I remember after one fight I got stitched up in a locker room by a guy who had Tourette's syndrome. In order to keep his hands from shaking, he had to let a steady stream of cusswords out of his mouth. *Shit, fuck, honey, fuck, Love ya Honey!* He said these over and over as he dug a needle into my skin. He actually turned out to be a quite capable stitch man, but this is what you'll find in the smaller promotions—a capable Tourette's guy who has to curse like a sailor to make sure he doesn't stitch something that vaguely looks like the state of Texas into your face. As a matter of fact, don't expect to get treated at all. If you were like me when I first started out and don't have the money to visit your local emergency room, it's possible to stitch up a cut yourself using Super Glue, which was originally developed for this exact purpose. To apply these "ghetto stitches," wipe the blood away from the laceration, pinch the wound shut with the fingers of one hand, and then apply a small dab of Super Glue across the seam using a Q-tip. Chances are the scar won't be very aesthetically pleasing, especially if the cut was deep and you needed stitches inside, but when you're broke as fuck, sometimes you got to go ghetto.

Best Techniques for Opening Cuts
(All Legal in MMA Competition—i.e., Wins Fights)

- Over-the-top elbow
- Grazing punch with leather gloves
- Knee to the face
- Side elbow from mount or guard

Chicken Soup for Your Scrotum
(A Word on Confidence)

Personally, I had very little confidence when I first began fighting, but, thank-fully, I had a secret ingredient that eliminated its importance—I didn't give a fuck about the consequences. Losing was fine by me as long as I got to hit some-one in the face. To me, that was exciting and fun. However, at the time I was living a "*Logan's Run* Lifestyle." If you've never seen the movie *Logan's Run*, it's about an idyllic future society where everyone is as happy as can be, but at the age of thirty they get sent to the "happy place," which in reality is a dog-food factory or some shit. I truly thought that I wouldn't make it past thirty, so what did I give a shit about a few teeth or a joint or two. This "give a shit" attitude is an excellent replacement for a complete lack of confidence, but just as it happened for me, it gets ripped out from underneath you at the age of twenty-nine. If you haven't built at least a little confidence by that time, you're pretty much screwed.

But self-help books are not the way to go (this book notwithstanding). Personally, I feel they are ruining America. They're evil for two reasons: they only make you feel worse about yourself, they are a colossal waste of time, and they cost a shitload of money (see how I put three reasons instead of two—ultramanly). If you feel the need to purchase a self-help book as a result of a lack of confidence, you are overcomplicating matters. All you need to do is find the root of the problem and take care of it. It seems so simple, but everywhere I go people try to suggest a self-help book, like the guy who works at the local Subway. He's a huge Tony Robbins freak, and every time I go to buy a sand-wich, he tells me about some new self-improvement book he purchased and how it changed his life. I feel like telling him, "Dude, you work in a Subway." Instead of reading a dozen self-help books and gleaning, at best, one or two useful hints, take a more analytical approach.

This is what I did in high school. Like most fifteen- or sixteen-year-old kids, I spent all my time hanging out in my room listening to Nine Inch Nails and cutting myself (that's what the songs say to do, right?). I went to a Catholic school where the girls wore ponytails and paraded around in come-fuck-me plaid skirts, but I lacked the self-confidence and articulation (not sure if that's a word) to talk to them. Senior year, I finally got fed up with being an awkward, uncomfortable kid. If I had gone the self-help-book route, I would probably still be fucked up today, but instead I started to fake confidence. Surprisingly enough, it worked. The more I faked it, the more confident I became. It was kind of like that game you play in a bar—you know, the one where you try to collect ten phone numbers. It doesn't matter if you talk to ten women and get shot down ten times, it only gets easier. When I went to college a few years later, everyone was sort of uncomfortable, but I wasn't, and I started having decent success with the ladies. It was kind of like I had willed it to happen. Moral of the story: fake it.

You May Have ZERO Self-Confidence If . . .

1)   . . . you plan your after-party at the emergency room. (Although I've never done this, I did have an after-party in the hospital after I fought Stephan Bonnar. Stephan's girlfriend picked up some McDonald's and Rory purchased some beers. When they walked in, Stephan and me were sitting next to each other. It was quite fun.)

2)   . . . you don't pee before a fight because you don't want to get discouraged by your small pecker.

3)   . . . you titter nervously in your corner, giggling uncontrollably and covering your mouth with your hand like a little girl.

4)   . . . your eyes fill up with tears during the announcements of the fighters.

Make the Extraordinary Ordinary
(Get in the Zone)

Someone a lot smarter than me talked about the importance of making the extraordinary ordinary. I have no clue who that somebody was because apparently I was born punch-drunk, but it is an excellent aspiration. Fighting, I suppose, can be classified as extraordinary because it triggers something in the brain and causes chemicals to be released into the body. Again, not sure what those chemicals are—adrenaline, estrogen, Neosporin, who the fuck knows. All I know for sure is that conceptually, when you walk down that aisle under those lights, and then climb into a cage to perform in front of thousands of screaming people and dozens of cameras, it's pretty fucking extraordinary.

For guys like Michael Jordan and Anderson Silva who've somehow found a way to unequivocally get the best of their opponents in their respective sports, it's just another day at the park—another game to win. For them, it's the *losing* that's extraordinary, 'cause neither does a lot of it. But us mere mortals tend to get nervous, and that nervousness tends to affect us in negative ways. Your heart starts beating wildly, you can't catch your breath, and your balls tingle. And don't forget about those chemicals—all that Astroturf and kerosene floating around through your veins will jack you up big-time. While the Jordans and Silvas (the *Anderson* Silvas—not to be confused with every other person in Brazil) of the world may be few and far between in terms of their athletic ability, it definitely pays to aspire to the way they approach the game. Try to make the extraordinary moments seem as ordinary as possible. And start simple: for example, figure out what warmup routine you want to do right before the fight, and then do that routine each day leading up to the bout. Your environment and the people around you will be different when you do the routine *on* fight day, but at least you can take shelter in the routine itself. It helps make the upcoming scrap seem more like practice and less like a pivotal moment in your life. When I was a coach on *The Ultimate Fighter,* I used a similar tactic on my guys. If one of them had a fight the following day, I'd throw on his entrance music and have him walk to the cage, take off his shirt, and then do three rounds of shadowboxing. The goal wasn't for him to improve techniquewise, but rather to get him comfortable with the whole process so it was less jarring on him the following day.

At the same time, you don't ever want to get to the point of being devoid of emotion altogether. Retain the excitement, but become familiar enough with your surroundings that you have perspective. This all comes with doing your homework and establishing a game plan about which you're confident. Striking a balance between ordinary and extraordinary is what musicians do all the time. They rehearse enough so that playing a song becomes instinctive, but they don't play a tune *so* much that it becomes stale in performance. (A note to my former roommate—you know who you are: fuck you for making me hate a-ha—I used to love that band before you played that goddamn "Take on me" into oblivion, dick.) Believe me, holding on to the excitement that anticipation offers is so important—that wash of emotion doesn't last forever, and when it fades, I'm sure you'd give just about anything to get it back.

Plan B Isn't Just a Morning-After

I feel it is important to have a backup plan both in fighting and in life. It can even be good to have a Plan C, Plan D, and Plan E. You don't want to think about these plans on a daily basis because that would take your focus away from Plan A, but you want to come up with a few and tuck them away in the back of your mind—an "Oh Shit" list for when you find yourself in a downward spiral. After all, it can be hard to find the perfect game plan your first time around. I love jujitsu so much because more than in other martial arts, the diversity of moves and locks affords you the opportunity to develop secondary and even tertiary strategies—you go for a *kimura* (chicken-winging the guy and cuffing his arm behind his back), and if it doesn't work, you go for an armbar (i.e., creating a joint where there is none and forcing the arm in the opposite direction) on the opposite side. If the armbar doesn't work, then you maybe try a guillotine choke (need I explain that one?) or go back to the *kimura*. You keep cycling through things so that you're never lost and hopeless and, eventually, you *will* find *some* game plan that does work.

Here's a personal anecdote to illustrate a life lesson. (You bought the book, so presumably you want to know something about me—*besides* my cup size, freak.) My plan was to be a professional MMA fighter. I trained my ass off for a number of years and competed in as many shows as possible, but I was stuck in the smaller promotions, which, surprise fucking surprise, resulted in a serious lack of funds. At times, I didn't make enough to put food on the table. It was rough going, and I probably would have tried something new had I not read the book *An Actor Prepares* by Konstantin Stanislavsky. Although the book, nay, *bible* (some self-help guides fall into the category of "biblical"—that's the exception to my no-self-help-guides rule) primarily gives advice on how to *act*, the author offers one really cool story about how a group of pirates used to jettison and then destroy their life rafts before going into battle, destroying any escape route. It seemed like a pretty smart tactic because every last pirate fought his ass off. I mean, what other choice did they have? Either they destroyed the enemy ship or they died trying.

Stanislavsky's telling made it seem like a truly awesome tactic that I should apply to my life, so that is what I did. I told myself that no matter how destitute I became, I would not give up on fighting. I did everything I could in training to excel in the sport. But then I suffered a rather severe injury back in 2004, when I took on Edson Pardue in the *Heat Fighting Championships 2* down in Brazil. Toward the beginning of the fight, he threw a leg kick and I dropped my left arm to block it. I felt a burst of pain in my forearm, but I forgot about it as he pummeled me repeatedly in the face. A few minutes later, I knocked him out with a hard right hand. After the fight, the pain in my arm set in. Adrenaline, piss, and vinegar can numb an injury in the heat of a fight, but that numbness doesn't last for long.

I went to the emergency room in Brazil, which turned out to be an experience in itself. First off, everyone was sitting on the floor. There were a bunch of chairs open, so immediately I thought, *FOOLS!* I jumped into a seat before anyone could snatch it away, but just before I made contact, I realized why it was vacant—it was filled with vomit. Growing frustrated, the promoter of the fight went to the front desk and bribed the receptionist so I could be seen more quickly. They took me in the back, and soon I was visted by this Indian lady that spoke with a British accent. She appeared quite intelligent, which pleased me because I knew I would get proper treatment. She took some X-rays, told me my arm was broken, and then called in someone to fix it. The guy that entered the room did not appear nearly as intelligent as the doctor. He was a big, burly guy in overalls who looked like he laid bricks during the day. I looked around for the smart Indian lady, but she was nowhere in sight. I was terrified, but without many options, I let this guy get busy on my arm. When he finished, I had this massive cast that looked like a two-year-old kid had gone nuts with papier-mâché.

The instant I returned to America, I went back to the doctor and was informed that the break was rather severe and I needed surgery to implant a steel plate. My choice of profession had left me without insurance or money (sometimes, my purses were five figures—with a decimal point right after the third), making the proposed surgery out of the question. And, on top of my not being able to fight, my broken arm also cost me my job as a bouncer.

It wasn't a lack of drive that caused me to say, "Enough is enough," but when you find yourself at risk of going hungry—and I don't mean living-in-a-tight-studio-and-chowing-down-on-lentil-soup-nightly hungry, I mean, skipping-breakfast-and-lunch-so-that-you-can-*afford*-that-nightly-can-of-lentil-soup hungry—you've gotta have a Plan B to go to, which, for me, was *be a cop*. And my Plan C was to go back to fighting. (That was about as far in the alphabet as I could get at that point, so there was no Plan D—now I can almost get to *Z* without singing the song.) I kept the dream alive in my head, so when I heard about the first *Ultimate Fighter* television show, I sent in an application. The rest you might have seen . . . Probably not.

If I had truly jettisoned all life rafts and stuck with fighting when I broke my arm, I have no idea where I would have ended up. It's possible that I could still be stuck in the smaller shows, pissed off at the world because I failed to make anything of my dream. Who knows? But a Plan B should not be an excuse to give up. That's the danger with creating a Plan B—reverting to it too early. You have to be honest with yourself—are you abandoning your dream because you realize you've hit rock bottom (you look like Christian Bale in *The Machinist*) or are you simply quitting because things have become too hard (your boss yelled at you and made you cry)? This is a question you have to answer, and if you are unable to answer it *honestly,* you might as well jettison the life rafts (i.e., have plans that go so deep into the alphabet you find yourself in double letters and numbers) because you'll most likely quit everything before you give yourself a chance to succeed. My advice: don't think of Plan B as giving up—just think of it as a modification of Plan A.

Love What You Do
(and Who You Are Doing)

A lot of people ask me why I fight, and the answer is pretty simple: I see mixed martial arts as the ultimate form of competition. If you're a hockey or football buff, you might disagree with me. After all, both sports are competitive and oftentimes violent. But what do the players from either sport do when they can't

settle a dispute on the field? They don't challenge the person they have a problem with to a race or a goal-shooting contest. No, they rip off their gear and
throw down. Why? Because fighting is the ultimate form of competition. If you
get beat in Ping-Pong or darts or basketball, you can always save face by saying,
"Well, I could still kick his ass." If you lose in fighting, you simply got beat.
Never once will you hear a fighter say, "He might have beat me in the cage, but
I would slaughter him in shuffleboard."

I enjoy a lot of sports, but fighting is by far the most gratifying because it
allows you to skip all the nonsense. Back when I was a cop, I made twenty-six
thousand a year. Fighting was always on my mind, and I told myself that if I
could pull in twenty-six thousand by stepping into the cage, I would give up the
badge and take up fighting full-time. I had no hope of someday making six figures per fight because, at the time, the sport was scraping by on the underground
and showing no signs of gaining in popularity. Even now, making considerably
more than twenty-six thousand a year, I live below my means because it makes
what I do seem less like a job and more like a passion. I purchase a new car approximately once every five years, and I spend roughly fifteen thousand dollars. It has been crashed into three times, and on each occasion I didn't even
ask the other driver for his insurance papers. If I had purchased a hundred-
thousand-dollar car and a bunch of other fancy shit I don't need, the bills
would pile up and fighting would seem more like a job and less like a passion. I
don't want to make any connections that will take away from what I love to do,
which is punching other people in the face. There. I said it.

I don't think there are right reasons and wrong reasons to fight—I just
think there are different reasons. If you get into MMA because you want to have
an excuse to get a bunch of tattoos and pick up floozies, hey, as long as it makes
you happy, why the hell not? If you climb into the cage because you clamor for
an organized, *legal* way to hurt people, more power to you, you fucking sicko.
With MMA having exploded on a global level, I'm sure there are guys out there
fighting for every reason under the sun. Regardless, as Ben Franklin said, "If
you get a job you love, you'll never work a day in your life." Me and ol' Ben Frank
would have been homeboys.

Underdoggy Style

If you're one of those guys who bounces around all the time happy as shit, I hate you. In addition to annoying chronically cynical guys like me, you're also screwing yourself in the long run because you create expectations. The first time you have a bad day, people will be like, "Oh, what's wrong with you? You need a tampon?" Fucking annoying. Trust me, you don't ever want people to expect anything from you, and the best way to accomplish that is to consciously calm yourself down when you're too fucking bubbly. It also doesn't hurt to have a healthy smattering of self-hate. If you've read the book sequentially and you're not all ADD'd out, skipping around the pages 'n shit, you've probably already got this down, but just to reiterate, maintain an even temper. The villain is always cackling away like he's got a hard-on and is relishing this dirty little secret he has with himself. The hero—Rocky, Daniel, Alex Grady (a word to the wise, check out *Best of the Best*)—is stone-faced, calculating, relatable-to. If you're an underdog, as long as you fight your ass off, people will be pleased with your performance, win or lose. Let me just tell you, if you are the favorite and lose, you basically become a heel overnight. (Come to think of it, I'd better check the odds on my next fight . . .) I don't care how confident you are that you can kick the shit out of your opponent, you never want to tip your hand. I'm not saying that you have to be tense and pissed off all the time. You should still relax and have fun in life; you just don't want to say or do things that will generate expectations. For example, if you tell a chick you have a massive schlong, she's probably going to be disappointed when you take your pants off. After all, women have an entirely different definition of massive. Once that word is mentioned, they start picturing things like the Leaning Tower of Pisa. However, if you tell a chick to judge for herself, when she takes your pants off and discovers an average-size meat stick, there's a 50 percent chance she won't be as disappointed.

Live Johnny Dangerously

There are two excellent ways to get injured in a fight. The first way is to step into the cage thinking you're going to get hurt. This mind-set, which we will call the pussy mind-set, is usually due to a severe lack of confidence, and although

I don't exactly know why, you're prophecy will usually become a reality. The second way is to go into a fight thinking there is no possible way in hell you can get hurt. This mind-set, which we'll call the king-of-crazy-fathers-never-let-your-daughters-near-this-cretin mind-set, is usually a by-product of a bloated confidence, and I've seen many "ain't no way he can hurt me" douche bags get carted away in an ambulance. If you're a fighter, for the sake of your longevity in the sport, try to be somewhere in the middle. But this also goes for people who do *anything* dangerous for a living and for thrill seekers. Realize there is danger in what you're doing and map out the quickest route to the hospital (which you will have well researched—a list of ethnic doctors on staff not named Forrest or Griffin is usually a good sign), but don't dwell on it. If you're dwelling on it, rethink your profession. Stage fright is natural until you start puking your guts out before the big monologue.

Be Passionate
(Just Don't Go Humping Your Opponent's Leg in the Half Guard Because That Definitely . . . Ain't . . . Cool)

I'm sending this one out to the fighters, but much of this philosophy applies to everyone. You'll never be great at something you half-ass, and this is *especially* true in fighting. If you want to reach the top of the MMA mountain, you've got to have a pretty intense passion for scrapping in the cage. When you're tired and beat up, going to the gym can be worse than going to the dentist. Such days suck in a major way, but you've got to bounce back. True success in MMA cannot be attained without a passion for resiliency, which is tantamount to being passionate for the sport. If you really feel the excitement waning (and you can tell this easily by how you approach the day you're scheduled to do your favorite training exercise—if you're a stand-up guy, and you're dreading boxing practice, chances are you're burning out), I recommend taking some time off. This is what happened to me—sort of. I was actually forced by a shoulder injury to take seven months off. But, in many ways, it was fortunate because I was so overtrained I could no longer protect myself. I still loved fighting, but my body and mind needed a break. Two months into the layoff, I was climbing the walls. Figuratively speaking. My shoulder wasn't gonna let me climb shit. But the break was a mixed blessing, because it made me realize just how important training and fighting had become in my life. When I finally returned to the gym, my passion had grown tenfold.

Close Your Piehole and Open Your Mind

When you think of all the different techniques that can be utilized in MMA competition, it is mind-boggling. There is always something new to learn, so if you think or behave like a know-it-all, you're, clinically speaking, pretty much retarded. I don't care if you're the best Brazilian jujitsu practitioner on the planet—there are all sorts of people out there who can show you new techniques and approaches.

In order to keep up with the rapid evolution of the sport, you've got to keep an open mind. A few years ago, I would have told you that there was no way in hell crazy karate kicks would work in the Octagon. Lyoto Machida made me feel foolish. The best way to grow as a fighter or as anything else is to keep your mouth closed and your mind open. Absorb all you can, keep what works, and throw out what, for you, doesn't. HOWEVER, once you get about six weeks out from a fight, it's time to close the doors to new techniques. The last month before a fight is not the time to learn new tricks—it's the time to hone the skills you already have.

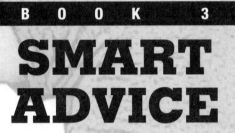

BOOK 3

SMART ADVICE

A Few Words on Clubbing

Is That Real Velvet?

After training hard all week, it's nice to blow off a little steam at the clubs. But when you live in a city like Las Vegas, trying to get into one of the more popular nightclubs can be as difficult as getting past White House security. But there are a few things you can do to make admittance easier.

1) *Become famous.* **And when I say famous, I do not mean reality show, Sanjaya what's-his-name famous. My stint on *The Ultimate Fighter* did dick fuck-all to impress bouncers. You've got to become Robert De Niro or Al Pacino famous.**

2) *Become rich.* **Or at least feign it. Slipping a ten spot to the bouncer and winking won't cut it. As a matter of fact, he might decide to clean the curb with your face out of principle. After all, he spent years neglecting to go to school and pumping roids into his swollen glutes to get this elevated position, and there is no way he'll let some honest Joe insult him with ten hard-earned dollars (and he'll be damned if he'll let you get away with that wink, sister). So unless you're ready to drop some serious cash, don't bother with the bribes.**

3) *Befriending a group of really hot chicks.** **Hot chicks always get into the clubs, and usually they're allowed to bring one or two guys with them. However, there is a strict three-to-one ratio. For every three hot chicks, one ugly dork is allowed in. If you've managed to befriend a bevy of chicks who have other**

---

*If you actually know and/or can hook up with that many hot chicks and have breached the friend zone, it is a much more direct and substantially cheaper evening to simply grab some Cuervo 1800 and a case of the High Life and drink beers while your new girlfriends do body shots off one another. Just turn on a little stripper music, keep promising that you'll all go to the club after you get your buzz going, and enjoy your own *personal* nightclub.

guy friends tagging along, go into sabotage mode. For exam-ple, whisper things like, "Your friend Bob, there. He seems pretty cool. I have no idea why he thinks your ass is fat." This strategy can work in the long term, but shit where you eat and you risk losing your bank, so try staying in the "friend zone."

4) *Join your local MMA gym.* The majority of bouncers are aspir-ing fighters, and if you constantly compliment them on their badassness during training, chances are they will let you into their club. Given that most bouncers are walking around at 220 or more, if you're a featherweight, and you're *not* Urijah Faber, the kiss-ass method is your best shot. But if you size up well with Mr. Pumpy Melons, the beat-the-living-piss-out-of-him-in-front-of-the-whole-gym-and-then-offer-to-buy-him-a-beer-afterward approach is a good one. This will earn you both his respect and friendship. However, I feel the urge to reiterate, *please* realistically assess your skills prior to at-tempting this method. In the worst-case scenario, not only does roid-rage bouncer boy displace your nose, he nicknames you "Pussy Boy," and no one named Pussy Boy is getting into his club.

5) *Join your local Gold's gym and seek out the biggest douche bag in the place.* If MMA frightens you and simply the *thought* of joining an MMA gym makes urine dribble down your thigh, I don't know why you're reading this. Hell, I don't even know how you know who *I* am. But, so as not to mix up the balls-y and the nutless, here is some advice for you timid folk. If, on your mission (I can't believe I'm treating Pussy Boy like Ethan Hunt) you hone in on a guy who clearly gelled his hair back before he came to work out or, if you're able to get close enough to some dude who smells like he just climbed out of a bottle of cologne (close enough means about twenty feet away, so don't worry about the guy thinking you're checking him out), he's probably a bouncer at a club. Introduce yourself, and over the next few weeks, rush to his aid whenever he needs a spot. You won't necessarily be his best friend come Friday night, but he'll at least respect you and will most likely let you

through the door. Quid pro quo, bitches. Admission: since you read *this* far, I suppose I owe you some honesty. I was Pussy Boy. I used this method. I tried the first four methods and none panned out. I'd rather not get into it, but yes, I didn't just play a Gold's Gym bitch on TV. In fact, if not for the few friendships I struck up with bouncers at the local Gold's, I would have no clue what the inside of a Vegas club looked like.

6) The last way to get into a club is to be on "The List." The fancier clubs rent out tables for an exorbitant amount of money, and the douche bag that coughed up the bread gets to make a list for his table. I don't know how many times I've had a friend tell me I'm on The List, only to get to the club and have the bounce say, "Nope, not here. Move." You're left standing there looking like a grade-A ass hat. To prevent this from happening, you want to get verbal confirmation that there *is* in fact a List and that *you are* in fact on it. To do this, all you have to do is call the club and ask them. If they have no idea what you're talking about, you should immediately hunt down your asshole friend and kick his ass. I wish I had come up with the bright idea of calling the club on my own, but it was passed on to me by Mark Lamen, a jujitsu phenom. It has led me to believe that jujitsu practitioners have more common sense than true MMA guys.

Finding the Party (Using a Little Technique I Like to Call the Wile E. Coyote)

If you've passed muster and find yourself *in* a fancy club, it can sometimes be difficult to know how to proceed. After all, you spend most nights freezing your ass off on the curb out front. Instead of heading to the bar and paying twenty-seven dollars for a couple of beers, I suggest drinking prior to going out—meathead football-player wannabes (I imagine several of *you* fall into that category—hell, you're probably *proud* of it) call it "pregaming." Okay, so this isn't news to most of you, but I'm just getting started. To keep things going, once you're *in* the club, search for an empty glass, wash it out in the bathroom sink, and then scout out the busiest table you can find. With a smile on your face, ease into the mix and strike up meaningless conversation with a drunk guy.

The reason you want a drunk guy is that he will seldom realize that he doesn't have a clue who you are. After a few sentences, reach casually for the bottle sitting at their table and pour yourself a tall one. I'll admit here that I don't drink that often—I'm convinced alcohol shrinks my scrote and suffocates my single teste—but I've seen many slide into my table and use this technique with great success. They don't know me or anyone in my posse, but there they are, chugging away at our booze. Instead of getting upset, I admire them for it. If it's gay-sailor night, I'll even tip my hat.

Getting Your Tail Between *Her* Legs Is as Simple as Resembling a Baldwin Brother—or Even a Rip Taylor

Just like getting into the club, the best way to succeed in the chick department is to have a recognizable face. Like, *Hollywood* recognizable. Ever seen *Superhero Movie*? It's a piece of shit, but that guy Miles Fisher's imitation of Tom Cruise gave me goose bumps. If you resemble anyone famous, and I mean even *slightly* resemble Orlando, Brad, or, fan me down, Jude, arrange it so that your friends come up to you and pretend you're him. You're suddenly that guy (not *that* guy, just that guy—no one wants to be *that* guy). Have them ask for your autograph as if they're just some fans or simply tell them to make YOU the center of attention for the night (with the standing promise that you'll do the same for them next time). The flurry alone will draw the interest of said women. But the good looks are a bonus, so I've heard. The magnetism of fame is the true aphrodisiac. I know this for a fact because it happened to me in a bar in Augusta. MMA athletes aren't as popular as movie stars, by any means, and I ain't no Cary Grant in the looks department (at least when I forget to shave), but in this bar, there just so happened to be a lot of fight enthusiasts. Guys kept coming up to me to talk about fighting, and the chicks in the place took notice. The majority of them had never seen an MMA fight in their life, but that didn't stop them from approaching me with "come fuck me" eyes. If you don't know the look I'm talking about, sorry for rubbing it in. Anyway, my buddy Luke, who was sitting off to the side, later told me that he watched several of these women take off their wedding rings. I can understand them doing that shit for some guy in the movies they had drooled over since they were little girls, but a guy they had never even heard of before? For all they knew, I could be Joey Buttafuoco. At first, I loved the attention and was sizing up these women to see who would look best in my bathrobe, but then disappointment kicked in: *Women might not like the music of the band, but they will fuck the lead singer.* They didn't give a shit about me, and I'll be damned if I'm going to let some hot chick ride this ugly train just so she can tell people about it. But, cynical as it may seem, I definitely understood that if you get a little cult of influence going, you'll get laid for sure.

Me and a couple of teammates from the Hardcore Gym wanted to test this theory, so we rented a few video cameras and some lights, and then walked around town like we were part of a reality show. We even got a couple of guys to run around to random girls and have them sign official-looking waivers. Shocked? Good. That was my goal. We never actually did this, but I fantasized about doing just that and I *swear* chicks would've been up to our nuts.

Tired Attire

The first rule is not to dress like your friends. When chicks do it, it's cute. When guys do it, it's just wrong. But if you hang out with guys who are into the same shit as you, this can sometimes be difficult to manage. For example, when I was a cop I noticed that all cops wear pretty much the same thing when off duty. They wear jeans, combat boots, and really tacky flannel shirts or black T-shirts that they tuck in—jelly belly optional. And let's assume all your friends are fighters—or wannabe fighters—the last thing you want is to all roll into the club in matching Affliction T-shirts. Even if the shirts are all different, it doesn't matter—the fact that they're all Affliction is bad enough. To avoid getting stuck into the "poser dipshit" category, I like to dress like a hobo. (I said dress, not smell.) You've of course got to dress nice enough to get into the club, which might mean a collared shirt, but the shirt doesn't have to have a Prada logo or anything. To give you a picture of what I'm talking about, think about how Tyler Durden dressed in *Fight Club*. The collar is often enough for admittance (assuming you use the greasy-palm suggestions I gave you above). Resembling a squatter might *seem* detrimental to your pimping ability, but I find, on the contrary, the majority of the time it actually helps. They'll look at your friends, all of whom are clad in expensive clothing, and then look at you, covered in rags. Instead of assuming that you're the brokest guy in the group, they'll assume that you're the richest, or at least the most interesting. After all, only a guy with "fuck you" money would come to a club looking like a slob. Reverse psychology to a tee. And if it doesn't work, women have a soft spot for the socially challenged. I know this for a fact.

The Only Pickup Lines You'll Ever Need

1) **My friends over there were wondering if you liked me.**

2) **Just to get this out of the way, I'd like some sausage and eggs for breakfast.**

3) **Forrest: Do you work for UPS?**

   Hot Chick: No. Why?

   Forrest: Because I swear you were checking out my package.

   Hot Chick (titters): I was. Now ravish me, please. Call down the power of the ancient gods and ravish me pagan style, you beast of a man.

Thank *You,* Mike Damone

I had a lot of trouble with rejection back in high school, but then I saw the movie *Fast Times at Ridgemont High*. In one scene, the cool scalper guy, Mike Damone, was giving "womanly" advice to the geek. He said something like, "You don't care whether she comes, lays, stays, or prays." I felt like he was talking directly to me, and after I acquired that mind-set, I no longer had problems picking up chicks. The trick is not investing too much time or effort into any one girl. You need to harness the buckshot approach and go after volume. If you talk to enough women, one is bound to like you. That was the great thing about being on a reality TV show. Chicks didn't like me any more or any less, but I was *exposed* to a wide variety of women. So if I approached twenty of them in a bar, one was bound to think, *I saw this dork on TV, and he was actually kind of funny. I guess I should let him sleep with me.* It also really helps to have fun and be in a good mood. Being a brooding invert only works if you're rakishly handsome. Needless to say, it did not work for me in high school.

DICK IN A BOX

by Big John

As you've probably figured out by now, Forrest is not normal. Nothing he does is normal, and that includes picking up chicks. Back when he was a cop and just getting into fighting, hot chicks would sometimes approach him and ask him why he had chosen those two professions. The majority of the time, he'd answer the exact same way: "I used to get beat up a lot in high school, I have low self-esteem, and I have a really small penis." He would say this straight-faced, not even crack a hint of a smile. The woman would usually say something like, "Sorry to hear that," and then try to cut the conversation short. Before she could slink away into the crowd, Forrest would ask her politely if she might be able to take a look at his pecker and let him know if it was really as small as he thought. He'd nervously draw open his zipper, and then slowly pull it out. Now I'm not a homo or anything, but Griffin ain't got no little dick, especially for a white guy. Expecting to see a teeny-weenie, the chick would be utterly amazed. As a matter of fact, caught in Forrest's Jedi mind trick, she'd think it was the biggest pecker she had ever seen. Her face would light up and the conversation would suddenly get interesting. Now, I'm not suggesting using this approach, because you have to be two parts crazy to get away with it, as well as have a decent-size schlong, but it seemed to work out quite good for Forrest back in the day.

Try this . . .

The "passive pickup." Search the bar for a group of attractive women and then migrate to their general area. Instead of engaging them in conversation, wait until a guy comes up and hits on them. *When* he fails, casually look over to the woman he hit on and say, within earshot, "Man, I can't believe that didn't work," in a sarcastic tone to no one in particular. If she smiles, immediately begin talking about how lame the guy was. As you can see, this requires you to bash some poor sap who actually *had* the balls to make a move, but hey, it's a dog-eat-dog world. If she says nothing to you, play with your cell phone and order a drink. The number one rule when it comes to picking up chicks is to not give a flying fuck. Remember, we're all going to die and very little of what we do in this world matters.

All the Ladies in the House Say OOOOOoooo . . .

(I don't know if that's what they actually say, because I don't listen to them)

I know women spend a great deal of time reading *Cosmo* magazine in an attempt to figure out what guys want, but guys really aren't that complicated. If we want something, we usually tell you, either through words or actions. In order to make your man happy, all you have to do is pick up on the cues and then react to them accordingly. For example, if you pick up on the cue that your man wants some alone time, suck it up and, temporarily, be neglected. Honestly, it's as simple as that.

When it comes to dating fighters, my advice is simply not to do it. They are cheap, preoccupied, and think their career is the most important thing in the world, even though they make next to nothing. I know what you're thinking: *What if I just fuck a fighter?* Still, don't do it. Even if they don't give you a venereal disease, they will probably give you ringworm or staph. (Haven't you been reading this book? I can understand the dudes skipping around, but chicks, I thought, had more of an appreciation for narrative flow and literary nuance.)

The Definitive Definition That Defines a Douche Bag

One day, while I was supposed to be writing down some intelligent shit to put into this book, I took a cruise to the store and noticed all these stupid-ass numbers on the back of high-end cars—E46 M3, E83 X3, E320. None of the numbers made any sense, but it got me thinking about the people who can recite each car model and how much each costs. It took but a few seconds for me to classify them as major douche bags. Then I started thinking about other types of people who could fall into the douche-bag category. The list grew too long to put into this book, so I've only included the top six (if you're wondering, *Why six? Why not ten or fifty?,* you're a round-number-loving douche bag). If you happen to do any of the things that are on this list, I hate to say it, but you're grade-A, brother.

1) If you always buy a specific brand of hair-care product, such as a creme or gel, and refuse to use anything else, you're a smelly douche bag.

2) If you have a person who waxes you, and you're not a professional swimmer, you're an overflowing douche bag.

3) If you've driven a Hummer outside of the military, you're a sergeant douche bag. If you're a chick who drives a Hummer, you're a douche baguette.

4) If you do things to people while driving that you wouldn't do while standing in a line, you're a fucking douche bag. Airport lines don't count because pretty much everyone does foul shit at the airport. But if you do things driving that you wouldn't regularly do in a line, such as cut someone off or give him the bird, I fucking hate you. When I'm rolling around with my big, goofy, gangly ass, hip-hopping because one leg is shorter than the other, which makes me look like a seventies pimp with a severe case of polio, people don't tend to fuck with me. But in a car, man, everyone is so fucking tough. Could it be because I drive a beat-up Scion?

5) If you regularly carry condoms on you, you're a douche bag. Unless you're Chuck Liddell, you don't need to walk around with condoms. I mean, come on, really? You carry condoms?

6) If you've ever tried to pick up a chick in church, you're *not* a douche bag, but you're going to hell. It's admirable, but you're taking a trip south when your ticket is up.

Heal the World

When I was a young buck, I was a proud member of the Webelos, which is the Boy Scouts' version of Brownies. I loved the organization with all my heart, but

unfortunately I never advanced in rank. While in our sacred den one afternoon, I got involved in an ice war with a group of fellow Webelos. What began
as a minor skirmish quickly turned into a full-fledged battlefield. My opponents overturned a table and took refuge behind it. The crafty little fuckers
would grab a handful of ice, pop up from behind the table, and then pelt me
with all their might. By the time I could return fire, they had already ducked
down behind the table. Just as I was about to surrender, an idea occurred to me.
The cooler from which I was receiving my ammunition also contained several
cans of soda, and I figured that if I launched one of those cans at the cement
wall above my rivals' heads, it would explode like a bomb and shower them
with sticky pop. Never having been one to actually think things through, I did
just that. With a sinister smile on my face, I hurtled the can of pop at the cement
wall.

The can of soda did not hit the cement wall. A millisecond after the cold
metal container left my palm, the scoutmaster popped his head in the door to
scream, "Hey, what are you kids—" He didn't get to finish his sentence because
the can of soda crashed headlong into his face. An hour later, I was asked not
to return to Webelos, which was unfortunate. Apparently, no merit badges are
given for successfully tagging your scoutmaster in the face with a can of Dr
Pepper. All they do is ask for you to leave and not return. However, in the brief
span of time I served in the Webelos, I learned the importance of making the
world a better place. When we went to a campground, we not only picked up
our trash, but also the trash of the people before us. We always tried to leave a
place clearer than we found it. As an adult, I still have that philosophy.

**I Always Try to Live My Life So That My Positive Output Is Greater
Than My Negative Output. If You Have Been Raised by Monkeys and
Have No Clue How to Go About This, Here Are Some Hints**

1) *Volunteer to help those less fortunate.* Back in Augusta, Georgia, I volunteered four hours of my time at the Golden Harvest
Food Bank every Saturday. I did this for a period of two years.
In addition to making you feel warm and fuzzy inside, it's also
a great way to meet hot hippie chicks. Although I'm not crazy
about the dress, music, or body hair that comes with hippie

chicks, I like the fact that they are concerned about the environment. They are also very compassionate about your shortcomings. If you come entirely too soon, they are understanding. Or so I've heard. Volunteering also looks great on your résumé. I tell everyone I possibly can about how I helped out at the food bank. Hell, I'm even writing about it in my book fifteen years later. But the one thing I always fail to mention is that my charitable donation of time was way back in 1994. Since then, I haven't done dick. Does that matter? Hell no. Once you have that merit badge, no one can ever take it away. It's a lot like screwing a supermodel. It doesn't matter how repulsed she is when she wakes up with a screaming headache and finds you nestled up to her bosom the next morning. She did the deed, and that's all that counts.

2) *Pick up after yourself and others.* The reason I'm adamant about this one is that the Japanese do it, and we can't let those fuckers beat us. There could be thousands of them walking up and down the same street, and you won't find a single piece of trash. And if there is a piece of trash, those fuckers will pick it up and put it in their pocket until they can find a trash can. How many Americans do you know that will carry someone else's trash around in their pocket until they can find a proper home for it? Not one. It's virtually incomprehensible, and this is unsatisfactory. Tell everyone you know to begin picking up trash. If we're lucky, it will become a trend that sweeps the nation, and we'll defeat the Japanese once again!

3) *Drive courteously.* I've left this one for last because it is by far the most important. Seriously, don't cut people off. If someone needs to get into your lane, let him or her into your lane. If they saw the lane was going to end and sped up, that's different; you cut their ass off and give them the finger. But if they are just trying to get over, don't be a dick. It's not a contest. That one car length of lost distance is not going to make a difference in your life (unless, of course, you add it up exponentially,

DICK IN A BOX

by Big John

I feel the need to elaborate on Forrest's obsession with drivers being courteous. He made it sound as though if you cut him off, he would get angered. That is not the truth—he will try to kill you. Remember how I was telling you that there are two sides to Forrest—the happy-go-lucky Forrest and the scary Forrest? Well, asshole drivers bring out the dark side in him. One time, we were driving home after an awesome training session. Both of us were as happy as could be, and then some guy cut him off. Forrest went apeshit and chased the prick for two miles, all the way to the guy's apartment complex. Forrest pulled in behind him, jumped out of the car, and unleashed a verbal assault the likes of which I had never heard. I know Forrest pretty well, and I could tell he was gearing up for a fight, and so I said, "Forrest, get back into the car." Immediately he spun around and started going apeshit on me. "Don't use my motherfucking name! Don't you use my motherfucking name!" The only reason he wouldn't want me to use his name is if he was planning on seriously wounding the son of a bitch. I'm glad I did, because it obviously snapped some sense into him. He got back into the car, but instead of driving away normally, he backed all the way down the street so the guy couldn't get his license-plate number. So trust me, drive courteously. You never know when you're going to meet Forrest Griffin on the road.

and then it will probably make a pretty big difference, like at least a couple of days of your time, which could have been spent on doing cool shit like watching television, but you're not supposed to add it up like that). If people fucked with me less on the road, I would be a lot happier of a person. We all would. However, I don't always practice what I preach. While doing this interview on the phone with Erich, I'm reading my notes on this subject, drinking a cup of coffee, and driving sixty-five down the freeway/sidewalk while all the other cars are pretty much at a dead stop. I'm weaving in and out of traffic, endangering not just my life, but also the lives of all the

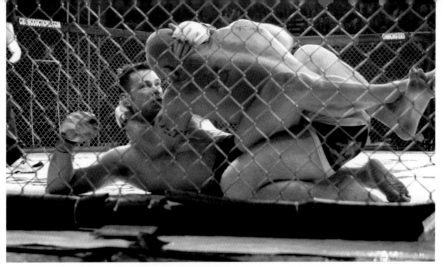

Attempting to strike Jeff Monson from my guard. (6/29/2002; photograph by Paul Thatcher)

Working to pass Jeff Monson's guard. (6/29/2002; photograph by Paul Thatcher)

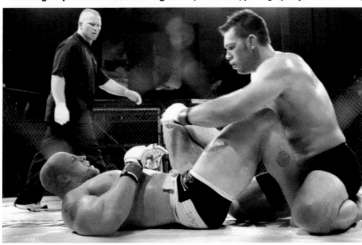

Earning a decision over Jeff Monson in WEFC 1. (6/19/2002; photograph by Paul Thatcher)

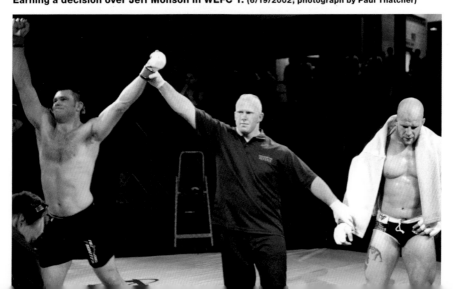

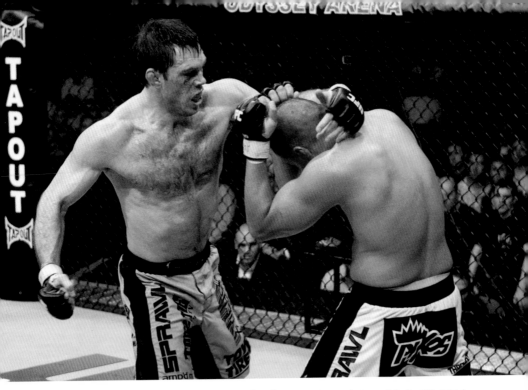

Working the dirty boxing clinch on Hector Ramirez. (6/16/2007; photograph by Paul Thatcher)

Landing a Thai kick to the ribs of Hector Ramirez. (6/16/2007; photograph by Paul Thatcher)

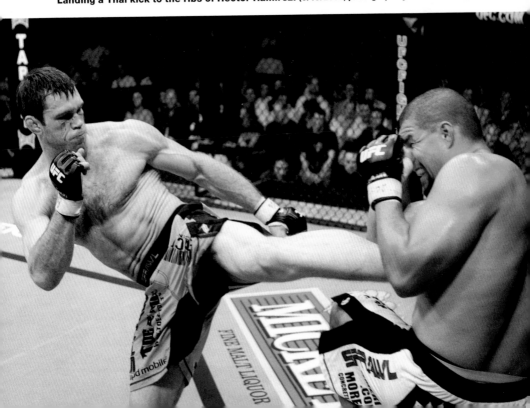

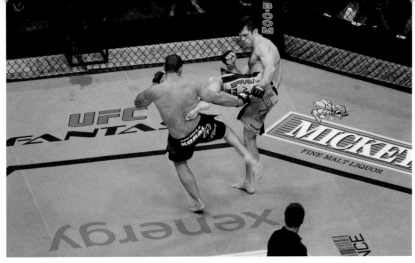

Landing a rib kick to Mauricio "Shogun" Rua. (9/22/2007; photograph by Paul Thatcher)

Working the ground 'n' pound on Rua. And what's up with using the small *n?* Are we really too lazy to spell out the word *and?* (9/22/2007; photograph by Paul Thatcher)

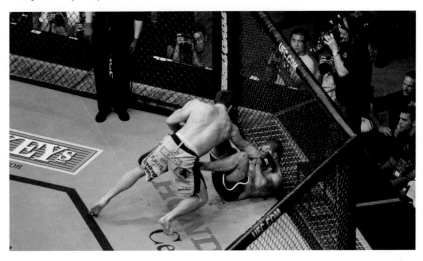

Finishing Rua off with a rear naked choke. (9/22/2007; photograph by Paul Thatcher)

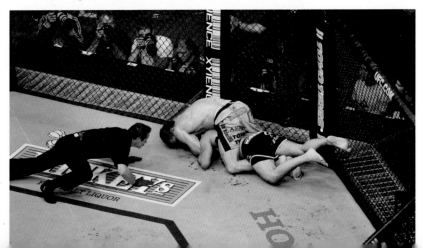

I'm attempting to capture Quinton Jackson in a guillotine choke. Meanwhile, the camera guy in the background is zoomed in on my ass. (7/5/2008; photograph by Paul Thatcher)

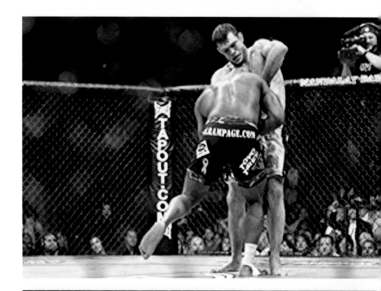

FORREST: ". . . and the waiter tells the jockey, 'So that's how I got the football stuck up my ass.'"

QUINTON: "You're killing me, Forrest. Tell me another, you're fucking killing me."
(7/5/2008; photograph by Paul Thatcher)

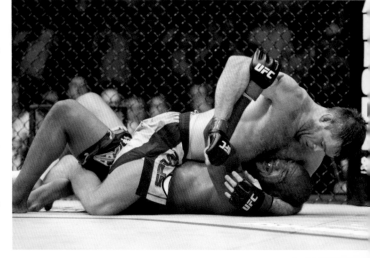

Say hello to my little friend.
(7/5/2008; photograph by Paul Thatcher)

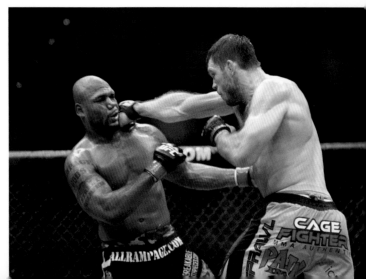

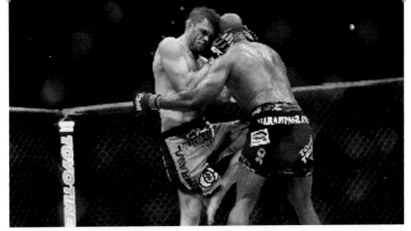

Although this looks suspiciously like the Good Ol' Fashioned Knee to the Nut Sac technique demonstrated in this book, I'm pretty sure this knee landed to Quinton's abdomen. (7/5/2008; photograph by Paul Thatcher)

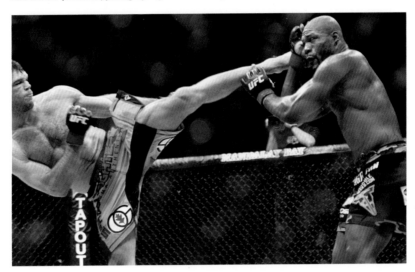

Attempting to damage Quinton's right arm with head kicks.
(7/5/2008; photograph by Paul Thatcher)

Getting hit by Quinton's right hand. (7/5/2008; photograph by Paul Thatcher)

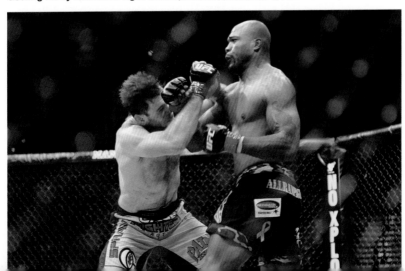

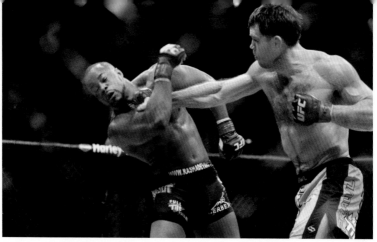

Tagging Rashad Evans with a hard right. (12/27/2008; photograph by Paul Thatcher)

OK, this is probably gonna hurt. (12/27/2008; photograph by Paul Thatcher)

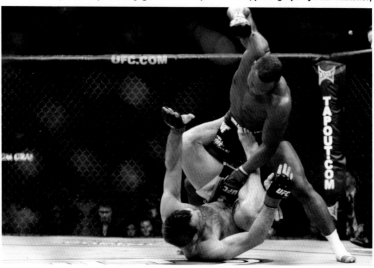

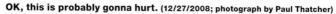

FORREST: ". . . and the waiter says to the jockey, 'So that's how I got the football stuck in my ass.'"

GRAY MAYNARD: "That's not cool, Forrest. Tend to your broken hand. I no longer want you to talk to me." (12/27/2008; photograph by Paul Thatcher)

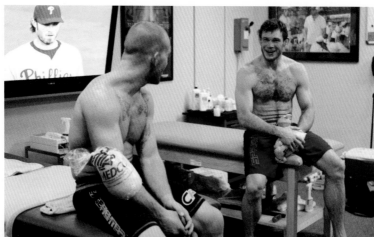

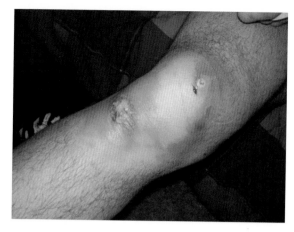

My nasty
case of staph.
(photograph
courtesy of the
author)

Adding to the ugly. (photograph courtesy of the author)

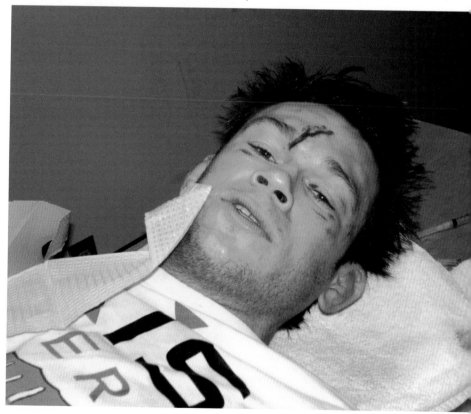

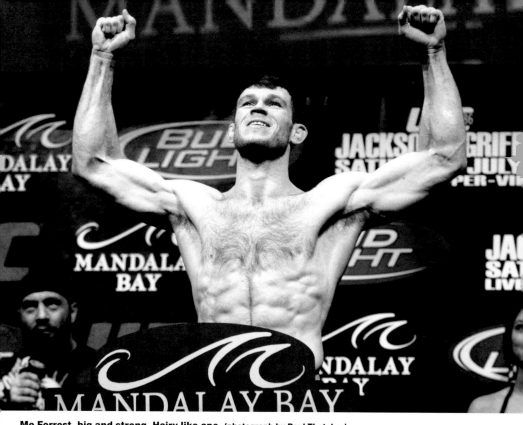

Me Forrest, big and strong. Hairy like ape. (photograph by Paul Thatcher)

"This is my rifle. There are many like it, but this one is mine . . ." (photograph courtesy of the author)

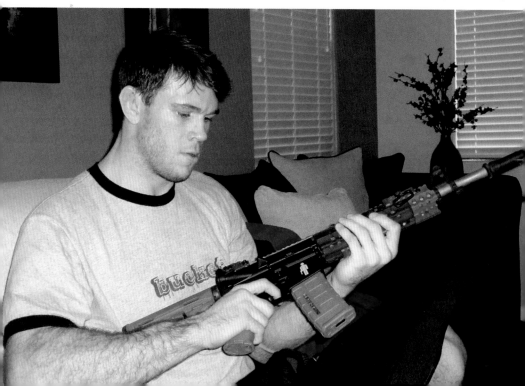

* * *

Further, Forrest forgot to mention the importance of being considerate to others. He's the most loyal guy I know, and he'll do just about anything for his friends, but at times he's lacking in the consideration department. For example, the night before he was to make his acting debut on *Law & Order*, I called him up and asked him if the show was appropriate for my three-year-old son to watch. I knew the show could get a little edgy, but with Forrest being my son's godfather and biggest hero, I didn't want him to miss out. Forrest's answer was this: "Of course it's okay for him to watch, dumb-ass."

The next night my son and me curl up on the couch in front of the TV. When Forrest's ugly mug appeared on the screen, my son was overwhelmed with happiness. He kept saying, "Forrest, Daddy. Forrest on the television." It was truly wonderful to see such joy and amazement in my son's eyes, and then out of nowhere, Forrest gets shot dead. My heart sunk, and an instant later my son starts screaming and crying. "Daddy, Forrest dead. Forrest dead," he kept repeating over and over. It took me twenty minutes to calm him down. It was a truly horrifying moment in my life that I blame entirely on Forrest's lack of consideration.

people around me, like those six kids in the back of the station wagon ahead of me. But I'm different. I mean, come on, I have a mental handicap.

The Right Woman Is *Not* Just a Swallow Away

If you plan on becoming a professional fighter, there are certain types of women you don't want to date. A lot of fighters won't give you this advice because they want to get laid, so they keep their options open. For them, the *wrong* woman can be the *right* woman—for an evening, anyway. But, having found the right woman, I have no fear of pissing off the opposite sex. So heed my words; just don't repeat them in public—only in the mirror. As a matter of fact, if one of the two chicks who actually read this book (earlier I had that number at three, but I was being optimistic) asks you what you thought about my advice on women, tell them this: "Forrest Griffin is a hermaphrodite piece of shit who hates his hairy vagina and takes it out on women." If you're foolish enough to agree with me, you'll most likely lose your spelunking privileges for at least a month. It's not that my advice is bad; it's just that women don't like men placing them into categories. There is, however, one exception to this rule. When chilling at the club with your old lady, you're allowed to point to the really hot chick getting all the attention and put *her* in a category—as long as that category is titled "slut" or "whore." This will usually prompt your woman to run at the mouth about the troglodyte in question for at least an hour, allowing you to ogle other hot chicks while she is preoccupied.

So what is the *wrong* kind of woman for a fighter? First and foremost, a girl that is with you simply *because* you're a fighter. They are sometimes masters at disguising their reasons, but there are telltale signs of a fighter fucker. For example, if she comes to every one of your training sessions and shouts things like "kick his fucking ass" while you are grappling, and then leaves a puddle of viscous fluid on the plastic visitor's chair when she gets up, she's probably got a fight fetish. I know what you are thinking: *That's fucking cool!* No, no, it's not. Fighters are usually unclean people who've had terrible childhoods. They're pretty much crazy people. If a chick dates fighters and fighters only, she, too, is probably pretty fucking crazy. She's the kind of chick who will dress like a megawhore to get attention, and then tell the guys who hit on her that you're going to beat the piss out of them. It doesn't matter if the perp has ten buddies guarding his back—she'll send you to slaughter by insulting their mothers and challenging them on your behalf. Chicks like that are into expensive cars and glamour and all that materialistic bullshit, and they'll most likely leave you the instant you lose your first fight. The *actual* author of this book, Erich Krauss, experienced this whorishness firsthand. Awhile back he cornered his friend Jason Pietz at an IFC event. After Jason kicked the living shit out of his opponent, the opponent's girlfriend approached him backstage and pretty much tried to blow him right there on the spot. I mean, come on. How fucked up does a girl have to be to try to blow the guy who just moments before bloodied up her boyfriend? Trust me, you do not want one of these skeezers. They can be fun in the sack with their fake tits, but these shallow, daddy-issue attention whores will put you through a living hell on a daily basis.*

But by the same token, you also don't want to go out with a woman who *detests* the fact that you fight. I can understand a woman's concern if you met her when you were working as a repairman and then, two years into the relationship, you decided to make the transition to MMA fighter. After all, fighters are not the nicest people to be around the month before a fight. The profession is a lot like bodybuilding—you're hungry all the time, sore all the time, and you generally feel like a sack of shit twenty-four hours a day, making you one moody son of a bitch. (If you love the woman you're with, you better make damn well sure fighting is a serious passion before making the transition because you very well might lose her.) But I'm talking about the kind of chick who *knows* you're a fighter when you meet her but waits until you're emotionally attached six months in to share her disdain for the sport and your involvement *in* it. If you detect that you're with this type of broad, immediately shed that dead skin. It doesn't matter if you were already considering giving up on the sport—no matter what new path you take, she will most likely have a problem with it. This is the type of woman who won't be happy until you have a chain around your neck and are following her every tug. It happened to a talented buddy of mine. He was a damn good fighter, but the chick he started dating gave him so much grief, he ended up walking away from the sport. He's a successful doctor now; what an idiot! He could be making 10 & 10 in the UFC.

Find a chick in the middle. One who doesn't hate the fact that you fight, but for whom the thought of you shattering another man's nose doesn't get her panties dripping wet. Although some things are better when they're extreme, women aren't one of them.

---

*Believe me, guys, and in all seriousness—you don't ever want to date a chick that is only into you because you are a fighter. Don't get me wrong, it may be fun as hell, but in the long run (and I know you won't listen to me and nor should you, because from what I hear, these chicks are freaks) you *will* suffer horribly.

DICK IN A BOX

by Luke

I don't know why Forrest is giving advice on the "right woman" because before he met his beautiful wife, his taste in the opposite sex was seriously demented. If we were at a county fair and I asked him to point out the hottest chick he could see, he wouldn't point to the supermodel in pumps and a tiny skirt. He would point to some backwater chick that had saggy tits and protruding tan lines. Seriously, he had some type of tanline fetish. A psychiatrist would probably read all sorts of stuff into this (and I think Forrest should see a psychiatrist at some point), but I know exactly how his strange taste in women developed. When we were kids and first discovered the hotness of girls, we went searching for porn. And where does one go searching for porn? In their dad's closets, of course. Well, instead of finding an issue of *Playboy* or *Penthouse* or *Hustler* in his father's hiding place, we discovered a pile of *EZ Rider* magazines. Now, I don't know if you have ever seen *EZ Rider,* but they often have half-naked chicks mounted on top of motorcycles or lifting their shirts at rallies. His pop was into bikes, so I'm pretty sure that's why he purchased the mags, but Forrest and I were looking at the chicks. Having never before seen naked women, we didn't have anything to use as a reference. We thought the chicks were all hot, when in fact they were all snaggle-toothed monsters. They had these massive bushes protruding out of

Warning Signs to Look out for with the Opposite Sex—in This Case, Opposite Sex Means Women (Nonfighters, Listen Up)

1) If on the first date a woman orders the most expensive thing on the menu and expects you to pay for it, she is a money grubber. Instead of paying the bill, tell her that her makeup is runny and send her to the bathroom to fix her face. If she takes her compact mirror but leaves her purse, steal her purse and sneak out the back door. If she takes her purse, order and consume the most expensive bottle of wine before bolting.

their stained panties, Frisbee-size nipples, boobs that sagged down to their waist, and, of course, tan lines.

Later in life, after I could adequately process our first adventure into porn, I realized that Forrest and me had been through a traumatic experience, not unlike two children who witness the slaughter of their parents. I was the strong one because I got over that day—I went on to become a healthy adult with a healthy view of beauty. Forrest was the weak one because he got stuck in that moment in time and went on thinking that tan lines and saggy boobs were attractive. When we'd head over the border to South Carolina as teenagers to visit the porn shops, I'd step up to the main rack that held the normal magazines. You know, *Playboy* and such. Forrest, however, would head to the seedy rack in the back of the store that held all the perverted specialty magazines. You know, like *Bush King* and *Tan Line Tatters.* I constantly hoped the phase would pass, but when he got girlfriends, they would all be these hippie chicks that worked in coffeehouses. They were nice and all that, but very few of them believed in bathing. I was worried about my friend for a long while, especially when he got famous. I thought he would either end up with a supermodel or a washed-up porn star. Luckily, he chose the supermodel.

2) If she asks you to buy her a dress or any type of jewelry on the first date, tell her that you will purchase it for her on your second date. Take her home and try to convince her to sleep with you—bring up the item she wanted you to buy as a bargaining chip. Whether she sleeps with you or not, conclude the evening by telling her that in fact there will *never* be a second date. Sounds mean, but don't forget who started it.

3) Steer clear of women who work in a bar or club that has an animal name. For example, "Spearmint Rhino," "Leopard Lounge," "Cheetahs." I just can't tell you that enough . . . you know

what, never mind. If you don't follow this, you *deserve* the
deep purple nipples.

4) If she talks about her ex-boyfriend and the size of his cock, immediately end the date. Immediately. However, later that evening you should call her mother and inform her that her
daughter is a whore. If the mother agrees and sounds hot, ask
her out on a date.

5) If on the first date she talks on the cell phone for more than a
minute, tell her that you're sorry for interrupting her and leave
Burger King immediately.

Fight Language You Need to Know
(or May God Have Mercy on Your Douche-Bag Soul)

Gameness: a willingness to fight anyone, anywhere, anytime, and in the back of
your mind, you know for a fact that you can win. This wonderful word origi-
nated from the training of pit bulls. If a pit bull is game, it has the will to fight
and kill its opponent. In order for a person to be game, he must have a mixture of toughness, heart, and stupidity. Even if he is getting his ass severely
stomped, he will never quit. He shows courage and determination even when
the end result might be catastrophic injury to himself. A perfect example of a
fighter who has gameness is Nick Diaz. Although he is a lightweight, he would
fight anyone from any weight class without thinking twice.

The numbers one through twenty: When you hear your opponent's cornermen
shout out the number two, they are not instructing their fighter to squat and
shit in the ring. The majority of the time, numbers represent a combination.
For example, the number two can represent a jab Thai kick. The number
three might represent a cross-knee Thai kick. Unless you have a spy in your
opponent's camp, it is impossible to tell what combination a particular number represents. However, when you hear a cornerman shouting numbers, it is
safe to assume that your opponent will shortly throw a combination.

Sprawl: The act of thrusting your hips toward the mat in an excited fashion.
There are only two occasions when a sprawl is called for: 1) when your opponent drops his elevation and shoots his body toward your legs to execute a

takedown; and 2) when an irate girlfriend throws a heavy object at your head. Sprawl is also a company that sends me a check on a regular basis for wearing their shorts . . . I know what you're thinking: *Forrest, you're not even good at sprawling, so why do you wear their shorts?* Well, because they don't have clothes that say cheesy shit, like "I'd rather be choking you out" or "Snap, Tap, or Nap." Personally, I don't like wearing clothes that invite confrontation.

Ground and pound: When someone refers to this word in a nonsexual sense, it means taking an opponent to the mat, obtaining a dominating top position, and then pulverizing his face with fists and elbows until his head looks like a six-month-old Halloween pumpkin.

Lay and pray: The art of taking an opponent down and lying on top of him in the hope of eking out a victory. Instead of throwing strikes and actually trying to win the fight, you want to sort of wiggle around on top of your opponent and give him as much man love as possible.

Check: The act of elevating your leg to block an opponent's kick. It's also a small piece of paper that you want to avoid touching when in a large group by running out of a restaurant or slipping off to a bathroom.

Jujitsu: When two sweaty people roll around together in pajamas or in shorts and no shirt. Just like when you played the spit game with your little brother in elementary school, the goal is to get your opponent to say uncle. However, instead of accomplishing this by hawking a loogy and dangling it toward your opponent's upturned face, you try your best to break his arms and legs and make him lose control of his bowels by choking him unconscious.

Glockenspiel: This hilarious word is actually the name of a musical instrument in the percussion family. It's a lot like a piano in that the keys are laid out next to one another, but the instrument is small enough for a fat German lady to strap it around her neck. This word is important because few people know what a glockenspiel is, and therefore it can be used as a size reference. For example, when a chick you want to take home inquires about the size of your cock, you can say, "Honey, my cock is as big as the keys on a glockenspiel." Sounds big, right? Well, what the subject probably won't know is that a glockenspiel has different size keys. The keys on one end are tiny, and the keys on the other end are large. If she gets angry and calls you a liar after sex,

DICK IN A BOX

by Big John

Forrest forgot to mention how insanity can sometimes be a good method for getting out of traffic tickets. I admit, this might not work for everyone, but somehow it worked for Forrest. While working as a bouncer, he got pulled over by a Clark County police officer for speeding. Normally he wouldn't care much about this, but in addition to being in a bad mood, his tags were expired, his driver's license was expired, and he didn't have insurance. This was about the same time he was living in that shitty, one-bedroom apartment, watching *Good Will Hunting* all day, and having imaginary conversations with me. Thinking that he would get hauled off to jail was more than he could take. When the officer approached his vehicle, instead of identifying himself as a former cop, like all men who have been in law enforcement would do, he began beating his head into the steering wheel of his shitty car. Now, Forrest has had some shitty cars, but this one was a serious piece of shit—the kind of car a homeless lady with four kids might live in. So you can only imagine what the cop was thinking. Here was this large, apparently deranged

pull out the picture of the glockenspiel that you carry in your wallet. In your case, the small key should already be circled.

Wretched: This is one of my favorite words, but unfortunately the only time it can be properly used is when someone farts, shits, et cetera . . .

Lassitude (noun): The art of lassoing small animals with a really thick rope: *her lassitude was amazing.*

What's Good for the Gray Goose Is Good for Your Gayness

Never ride on the subway reading a copy of the acclaimed novel *The Picture of Dorian Gray*. If you're not one to trust the advice of a complete stranger, I guess I'll tell you why. A while ago I made a trip to Washington, D.C., and had to get

individual, repeatedly bouncing his head off the steering wheel and crying like the day he was born. Naturally, the police officer asked him to stop. Forrest took his advice and stopped beating his head into the steering wheel, but apparently sitting there idly and answering the cop's questions wasn't an option. So Forrest exited the vehicle and began kicking the front left tire and pounding on the hood with his fists. Fearing for his life, the cop dropped his hand to his gun and ordered Forrest back into his car. Again, Forrest obeyed, but the instant he was back in the seat, he began to bite and chew on his steering wheel like a rabid dog. The cop attempted to ask Forrest a few questions, but when he received no answer, he dropped a business card for the county mental-health facility into Forrest's lap, slowly backed away to his squad car, and sped off. If Forrest had only mentioned that he was a former cop, he probably would have gotten off, but his antics led to a much more entertaining story for this book. It was one hell of a way to get out of a moving violation.

around by subway. Not wanting to engage in conversation with my fellow travelers, I pulled out the copy of *The Picture of Dorian Gray* that I had recently picked up, based upon a friend's recommendation. After reading a couple of pages, I noticed that a guy was standing above me, staring into my eyes with a smile on his face. It was obvious that he wanted more than my autograph, so I quickly dropped my eyes and pretended to keep reading. Eventually he went away and I got back into the story. I read maybe another two or three pages when I noticed another man standing above me, giving me that same look. Thinking that I was just being homophobic, I returned a smile and again continued to read. I noticed him leave in my peripheral vision, but he was replaced by another man with a warm smile.

Slightly freaked out at this point, I looked up at this guy and shook my head as if to say, "What?" His smile widened, his eyes narrowed seductively, and he nodded to the book I was holding. I flipped it over just to make sure the jacket didn't say *The Idiot's Guide to Man Love*. It still said *The Picture of Dorian Gray*, so I looked back at him and shrugged my shoulders. He flipped his head back, clearly insulted, and strutted off. Truly perplexed, I Googled the author, Oscar Wilde, when I got home, and learned that he was gay. I felt bad for the guy because I'm sure when he wrote the book over a hundred years prior, his intention wasn't for it to become a calling card for hot, gay sex. So heed my warning, if you read this book, do so in the privacy of your own home. Well, unless . . .

A Good Motto to Live By

If you're looking for a good motto to live by, look no further than the one I saw written on the wall of my local gun club: *As a good American, you should have a smile on your face and kind words for everyone you meet. As well as a plan to kill them.*

My Recommendations . . . Bitch

There's a good chance the majority of the horseshit advice I've given you in this book won't work, but the one thing I pride myself on is my taste in movies, television shows, and music. I am a pop-culture connoisseur. If you disagree with one of my recommendations, I don't need to meet you or talk to you on the phone to know your type. You're undoubtedly an inbred douche bag who regularly attends feltching parties. Nobody loves you or wants to be your friend. You're a loser. So go feltch someone, loser. Go sit your loser ass in a public restroom and feltch the guy in the stall next to you. Oh, and by the way, fuck you.

Movies

Grandma's Boy: This one is on the top of the list because it's the best movie eva—and I don't even smoke weed.

28 Days Later: This movie reinvented the horror genre by simply making the zombies move faster. I can just see the writers sitting around in a room, trying to come up with an angle that hasn't been done a zillion times. Suddenly one guy jumps up. "I got it, let's make them move superfast." If I had been in the meeting, I would have made this guy feel small with insults and then spit on his shoes. Shows you how much I know—they actually pulled it off.

Intacto: This movie is on the list because it is foreign. Yes, I'm one of those pompous assholes who likes to talk pretentiously about foreign films I can't understand in order to appear smarter and more cultured than I really am. But seriously, this movie is a delightful cinematic collage of sardonic humor and wit that enlightens the senses like an aged bottle of wine from the south of France.

Fear and Loathing in Las Vegas/Where the Buffalo Roam: These two movies are very similar because they're both based on the life of Hunter S. Thompson. They also both rock in a major way. I've been told it's best to watch them under the influence of a powerful hallucinogen, but this is certainly not mandatory. I've watched them both sober as a minister and they're still fuckin' awesome. In fact, I liked them so much I moved to Las Vegas. Seriously.

Unforgiven: This movie is slow and depressing, which is just how I like 'em. It's also how I like my women. Wait, that doesn't even make sense. Never mind . . . And damn straight I sip on cappuccino when I talk about my movies. I may even wear a beret. Do somethin'. (I'm not feeling quite right at this moment in time.)

Charade: This movie is more clever than any other movie ever.

Stranger Than Fiction: I should hate this movie because my wife told me that she would bail on me in a heartbeat for the main character, Harold Crick. If it was anything less than hilarious, I would have given it a thumbs-down. But I'll admit—if Harold Crick propositioned me, I would need at least a few minutes to think about it.

Good Will Hunting: For a two-year period in my life, I didn't have cable, and this was one of the two movies that I owned. I played it over and over for ambient noise, and after about a year, I actually believed that the main characters were my friends. I even began talking like them. How you like *them* apples, bitch?

Gladiator: This is the most awesome, manly movie since *Braveheart*. Great movie to watch before a fight.

Brick: This is one of the most original movies to come out in a long time. It's about awesomeness.

Caddyshack: This movie influenced the way we speak in modern times. I seriously don't understand how anyone could not like this movie—and that means you, Erich Krauss. Fucking retard.

Meatballs: Bill Murray's character, Tripper Harrison, is as cool as we all want to be. The movie is great.

Super Troopers: It's everything that being a cop should be, but isn't.

Fight Club: This movie actually ruined my life. Instead of taking it as a black comedy, I took it seriously. For the longest time I contemplated giving up all my worldly possessions and living like a Native American. But seriously, we all really should wear leather clothing because that shit lasts longer than cotton or spandex.

The Good, the Bad and the Ugly: The coauthor of this book, Erich Krauss, actually made me put this one on the list. I guess it's his *faaavorite* movie. When I told him I actually liked a *Fistful of Dollars* better, he almost began crying.

Once Upon a Time in the West: This movie should be seen by every guy because it shows you what true manliness is all about. It's slow, but give it a shot.

The Empire Strikes Back: The reason I picked this over the other *Star Wars* flicks is that I hate movies that have happy endings.

Bands

Nine Inch Nails: They got me through some dark, depressing times in high school . . . or maybe they just made those times darker. I still have scars on my arms that they're responsible for.

Guns n' Roses (circa 1987): No explanation needed.

Rolling Stones: They are actually a hundred and seven years old, and they still play better music than the rock bands today . . . I've heard that since they are senior citizens, they actually get a discount on their street drugs.

Nick Cave and the Bad Seeds: All their love songs are basically horror stories. How true is that?

T.I.: You know, "Got my nine in my left, a forty-five in my other hand . . ." You got to love a guy who gets arrested by the ATF for trying to purchase a machine gun.

DICK IN A BOX

by Big John

Although a lot of the shit Forrest says in this book might sound like a joke, the majority of it is real. That includes him talking like the guys from *Good Will Hunting*. Around the same time that he was having imaginary conversations with me, he watched that movie over and over maybe a thousand times. It didn't matter what time of the day or night you walked into his shitty, run-down apartment—*Good Will Hunting* would always be playing. For most people, playing the same movie nonstop would be a form of torture. I mean, isn't that what crazy scientists do to fuck with people's heads—play the same shit over and over until the subject loses any resemblance of a mind? I suggested that he purchase cable to get some variety, but Forrest hated regular TV. He also held the belief that cable was for pussies. He was perfectly content warping his mind with *Good Will Hunting*. But instead of going crazy like most people would, he became one of the characters in the movie. In addition to talking with a Boston accent, he would quote lines out of the movie. If he couldn't find a line in the movie that resembled what he wanted to say, he would pull shit from other movies (but keep the Boston accent). Just when I became certain that Forrest's speech had forever changed, the VHS tape broke from overuse. A short while later, his speech returned to normal.

TV Shows

Dexter: This show makes me want to kill people more than I already do. Don't worry, I know I'm not smart enough to get away with it.

Psych: This show is about cool, clever shit. I also have a non-gay-man crush on James Roday. Well, at least 95 percent nongay.

Firefly: The best TV show of all time.

Pushing Daisies: The best TV show of all time. This time I mean it. The fact that this show was canceled has caused me to lose all faith in humanity. If people cannot appreciate *Pushing Daisies,* we are doomed. What? They canceled it? Fuck.

A Gym by Any Other Name
Don't Smell as Sweet

If you're just getting into mixed martial arts, before worrying about finding a fight coach, a manager, and a decent promoter, you've got to put in at least a year of hard training. (How did I come up with a year? . . . Because I said so.) How quickly you advance will depend a lot on your natural athleticism and motivation, but it is also extremely important to find a good gym. Luckily, the majority of gyms allow you to take an introductory trial, and I strongly suggest going to as many of these as possible before making your decision. It's easy to get swayed by metals and trophies and titles, most of which belong to the gym's coaches, but oftentimes great fighters make horrible coaches. In the beginning, you don't need a world-champion jujitsu black belt. All you need is someone who will take the time to show you the basics, which can be accomplished by a blue belt. After each introductory class, you should ask yourself three things: 1) Did I have fun? 2) Did I get pushed? 3) Did I learn something? If the answer to these questions is yes, then you've probably found a good gym to kick-start your training. However, it is also important to take location into consideration. If the best gym is twenty minutes across town, there is a larger probability that you'll bail on class after a busy day. If you're like most of us and have motivational issues, sometimes your best bet is to choose the gym that is not *quite* as good but more convenient. Better to get to a decent gym three times a week than a great gym three times a month. Fatty.

Put Me in, Coach
(but Please Don't Push from Behind)

Once you make the decision to start fighting professionally, it's in your best interests to find a fight coach to monitor your training and prepare you for your upcoming bouts. I was fortunate because I began my training with a group of guys who were all active fighters, and when I showed promise in the sport, they unselfishly tailored practice to my needs. They also proved to be excellent cornermen, which often isn't the case. I've seen this a lot—a fighter agrees to corner his buddy and help him through weight cutting and all the bullshit he needs to do to get ready for the big night, but having just recently come off a fight himself, all he wants to do is party. When it comes to fight night, the cornerman is either hungover or still drunk, leading to predictably terrible advice. To avoid such an outcome, as well as get the best possible training leading up to the fight, it is in your best interest to get an actual fight coach.

There are a lot of fight coaches out there, but finding the right one can be difficult. Oftentimes, the right one isn't the best one. Take Greg Jackson, for example. The guy is undoubtedly one of the best coaches out there, but he's got more than a dozen professional fighters. Unless you're a UFC champion, he's going to give his other fighters priority. He'll give you excellent attention when it's your time, but the guy only has so many hours in the day, and if his schedule is overbooked, the smaller names get bumped from the roster. I've had opportunities to train with a number of top Muay Thai coaches, but the reason I remain with my coach is that I'M HIS PRIORITY (bigger name don't mean better). If something comes up in my schedule, he bumps the other guys to ensure I get my time with him. The primary thing to look for is attention.

Finding a coach also comes down to money. If you're like most fighters getting their start, you're dirt-poor, which means you can't afford to pay your coach an hourly rate. To get around this, a lot of fighters offer their coach 10 percent of their fighting purse. This can seem like a lot of money, but when you're competing in the smaller events making five hundred to show and five hundred to win, you're coach at best will make a hundred bucks. Considering the time he has to invest getting you ready for a fight, it boils down to pennies an hour. So in the beginning, the key is to find someone with a modicum of MMA knowledge who believes in you. It helps if they're independently wealthy, but that's not *your* problem.

As your rep grows, you'll have more options. You'll most likely get offers from some of the better-known coaches in the sport and leave poor Mickey— who had to survive on escarole soup in order to train your unappreciative ass—drowning in a puddle of his own tears. But if you wanna be a fighter, you've gotta get selfish and go with the best being offered to you. But as a warning, some of these coaches come attached to teams—meaning if you want Bill as your Muay Thai coach, you have to take João for jujitsu, Gary for boxing, and Tim for conditioning. They're like a private practice. Personally, I have chosen not to take this route. Being a part of a fight team has never appealed to me— I'm sort of a micromanager like that. I know my strengths and weaknesses and have a pretty good sense of what, together, will compose the best program for me. So I hire various coaches to help me with my training. I've got a jujitsu coach, a Muay Thai coach, a couple of boxing coaches, and then I use fellow fighter Mike Pyle to help me put my overall game plan together. That's just how I roll.

Finding a Fight Manager

Having a fight manager isn't mandatory, but it is certainly helpful, young fighters. "But, Forrest, I work at the gas station for three bucks an hour and you're a big famous fighter with lots of money and cute dimples." Okay, you got me. I do have cute dimples. But, even when I started out back in the day, I had a fight manager. His name was Frank Bishop, and he was basically a guy who got on the Internet and searched for promoters who had openings in their events. Once he found me a fight, he'd get the paperwork and forge my signature so I didn't have to drive all the way down to his office. That's about all he did. His only qualifications were that he could talk on the telephone and use a computer, but he prevented me from having to do a bunch of bullshit that would take time away from my training.

But just because you have a manager doesn't mean he'll be able to pull in big-money deals right off the bat. The biggest fight my first manager got me was with Dan Severn. I was supposed to receive two hundred and fifty bucks, but because of a misunderstanding, I only received two hundred. The bottom line is that if you want the money to start rolling in, you've got to win fights and make a name for yourself. Once you do that, the better-known managers will get drawn toward you like flies toward shit. Then, as you did with Mickey, you may have to leave your scrappy manager for greener pastures. For a small percentage of everything you make, a good manager will get you large fights,

DICK IN A BOX

by Adam Singer

I noticed that in the last section Forrest talked about the importance of having a sober cornerman, which is quite comical because every time he gets near a cage when he's not fighting, he's stone drunk. I remember one time not long ago he was asked to referee a cage fight in Macon, Georgia. Even though he was quite drunk at the time, he happily agreed. As it turned out, the fight was between a sixty-year-old man named Skip and a twenty-one-year-old kid. So Forrest climbed into the ring and started the action. A few seconds later, the twenty-one-year-old kid knocks the old man down, mounts him, and starts beating the living shit out of him with punches and elbows. Any referee in his right mind would have immediately stopped the action, but that's not what Forrest did. Squatting down, he began shouting, "Skip, it's up to you. It's up to you, Skip." Well, Skip didn't hear what Forrest was saying because he was unconscious at that point. The kid just kept dropping savage punches to

sponsorship deals, and free goods. They'll also fill out the mountains of paperwork and market you to the public. By nature, managers tend to be sleazy people. A good manager is still sleazy, he just isn't sleazy to you. However, regardless of *who* your manager is and what kind of golden rep he has, read everything you sign. I remember awhile back a promoter paid Din Thomas some money to keep him exclusive, but he never ended up seeing a penny of it. Around that same time, I had a few fights where the checks bounced. Managers tend to have an obsession with money, and it's best not to tempt them by putting all your finances in their hands.

Those Are My Cornermen You're Talking About

Before every fight, tell your corner how you want them to talk to you. Personally, I like calm, positive instruction. Having more than one person talking at a time confuses my simple mind. However, a lot of fighters like their corner-

Skip's face, and Forrest kept shouting, "It's up to you, Skip. It's up to you." Eventually, Skip woke up in the middle of the beating and tapped. It was the most horrific refereeing job I had ever seen, but that was pretty much run-of-the-mill for Forrest. He has actually been asked to referee a number of fights in Georgia, and generally he's done a terrible job each time. When it comes to cornering fighters, he's no better. I remember one time Forrest and me got shit-faced before cornering one of our amateur fighters. Just as our guy climbed into the cage, Forrest and me got into an argument about something. Instead of doing our job and giving our guy instructions, we spent the whole fight yelling at each other. Luckily, our boy slammed his opponent to the mat and finished him fairly quickly. I was pretty disgusted by the whole thing, so I settled our little dispute after the fight by palming Forrest as hard as I possibly could in the nuts while in the parking lot of a Steak 'n Shake . . . Ahhh, memories.

men to be a lot more confrontational. Some actually *like* them to shout degrading comments such as, "What are you doing, you pathetic puddle of panty waste? Why aren't you hitting him? Why aren't you kicking him? You're going to lose this fight and then you won't be nothing." And others like their cornermen to psych them up, no matter how poorly they're doing. They could be getting the shit kicked out of them and still want to hear things like, "He might have kicked you a dozen times in the face, but that ain't nothing. I think you hurt his shin with your skull. Look at him over there, smiling with your blood all over him. He's going to crack—any second now he's going to crack!" I'm not going to tell you what is the wrong approach because we all get motivated differently. The important part is realizing what approach works best for you, and then passing that information on to your cornermen before you're two rounds deep into a fight. You'd be surprised how important this is. When you're exhausted and beat up, the wrong words from those in your corner can make you want to quit or fight them, while the right ones can have a revitalizing effect. But also remember that you brought some of these

blockheads with you to the fight because you think they might have something valuable to offer. So, be ready to listen. The right coach should have
perspective and see where your opponent is weak so that he can tip you off.
You can gain valuable insight as the fight progresses. A fight is no time to lose
confidence in your cornermen.

42 FIGHTING TIPS

STANCE

Every martial art has different guidelines regarding stance, and those guidelines are set by the rules and goals of that particular style. In Greco-Roman wrestling, the goal is to chuck your opponent to the mat, but with the rules prohibiting you from dropping your hands below your opponent's waist, the majority of your techniques are executed from the clinch, making a high stance most appropriate to the style. In freestyle wrestling, the goal is also to take your opponent to the mat, but with the rules allowing you to attack his legs, assuming a low stance is often more effective. In Muay Thai, the goal is to bludgeon your opponent with strikes. As a result, a high stance is a must. Although the stance of two fighters from the same discipline might appear quite different, they both follow the same set of general guidelines. It is no different in MMA. In order to be effective in a sport where both striking and grappling are allowed, your stance must adhere to a set of guidelines. Your height, build, strengths, and weaknesses will determine the nuances of your stance, but breaking the general guidelines will create openings that your opponent can capitalize upon and likely lead to your demise.

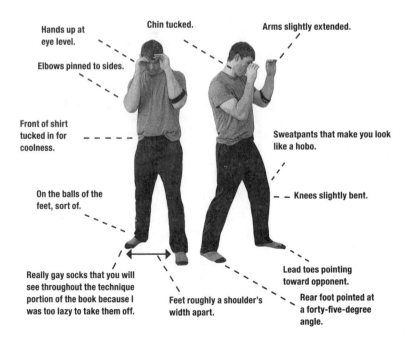

Hands up at eye level.

Chin tucked.

Arms slightly extended.

Elbows pinned to sides.

Front of shirt tucked in for coolness.

Sweatpants that make you look like a hobo.

On the balls of the feet, sort of.

Knees slightly bent.

Really gay socks that you will see throughout the technique portion of the book because I was too lazy to take them off.

Feet roughly a shoulder's width apart.

Lead toes pointing toward opponent.

Rear foot pointed at a forty-five-degree angle.

throbbing **TIP #1: FEET A SHOULDER'S WIDTH APART**

When you assume a fighting stance, your feet should be spread roughly a shoulder's width apart. In addition to providing a perfect blend of balance and mobility, this gives you a strong base, allowing you to effectively execute offensive and defensive techniques.

most likely infected **TIP #2: STRAIGHT AND FORTY-FIVE**

Foot positioning is very important. To maintain a proper stance, you want the toes of your lead foot pointing toward your opponent at all times and the toes of your rear foot pointing off to the side at a forty-five-degree angle. By positioning your feet in this manner, you can explode in any direction and maximize your offensive and defensive options.

veiny **TIP #3: BALLS OF YOUR FEET**

You never want to be flat-footed. If your heels are on the mat, you compromise your balance, hinder your ability to execute explosive attacks, and make it much more difficult to evade your opponent's attacks. For these reasons, you always want to remain on the balls of your feet.

I swear, honey, just the **TIP #4: KNEES SLIGHTLY BENT**

Always keep your knees slightly bent. Just as with remaining on the balls of your feet, this creates a spring effect, allowing you to attack or defend at the drop of a dime. If your knees are locked, your balance is compromised and your legs can easily be injured or broken by kicks or takedowns. However, it is important not to bend your knees too much, as this will make it difficult to strike or defend against strikes.

bulbous **TIP #5: HANDS UP BITCH**

This is the most important tip of the lot. By keeping your hands up at eye level, you create a barrier your opponent has to break through to reach your face. I know what you're thinking— *Forrest, I've seen you with your hands down by your waist in more than a few fights.* True, but I was born ugly, so I don't give a damn about busting up my mug. I'm not going to lie—keeping your hands up when fatigued can be a major son of a bitch. It can feel like you're holding two fifty-pound weights above your shoulders. If you absolutely can't hold them up any longer, use your feet; circle, backpedal, shake your arms out. But when you step back into striking range, return your hands to their proper positions, as they are the gatekeepers to your good looks.

smell my **TIP #6: ARMS SLIGHTLY EXTENDED**

In addition to keeping your arms up, you also want to keep them properly extended. If you hold them too close to your face, it can be difficult to utilize any form of blocking other than the boxing cover-up, which doesn't tend to work that well in MMA because of the smallness of the gloves. If you keep them extended too far away from your body, it can be difficult to strike with any type of real power—unless, of course, you have mastered Bruce Lee's one-inch punch. (For all you dumb-asses, that's called sarcasm.) The goal is to find that happy medium where you can both strike and defend against strikes effectively.

oh my God, is that your TIP #7: ELBOWS IN

Never let your elbows flare out to your sides. Keeping them tucked in when striking allows you to transfer the energy generated by your feet and hips through your arm and into your opponent. When in your stance, keeping your elbows tucked allows you to block strikes aimed at your body. If you forget this cardinal rule and let your elbows drift away from your sides, your opponent can use them as handles to pull you off balance and set up a takedown.

purple TIP #8: CHIN TUCKED AND SHOULDERS SHRUGGED

Whether you are fighting on your feet or off your back, keeping your chin tucked is mandatory. If you're the type of douche bag who needs to know reasons, let me offer you some: 1) It makes your head less of an empty ball bobbling on the end of a stick and more a part of your shoulders, which in turn protects your jaw from getting knocked to the back side of your dome by your opponent's fist. 2) If your opponent should heft you off your feet and execute a throw, keeping your chin tucked can prevent you from breaking that good ol' neck of yours. 3) When fighting off your back, it hinders your opponent from bouncing your head off the canvas like a basketball and causing you serious damage (as if head trauma could do you any worse). Although breaking this habit can be difficult, there are things you can do. During practice, pinch a tennis ball between your chin and chest while hitting the mitts, working on the heavy bag, and doing light sparring. At first the ball will most likely fall every two seconds, but with time your chin will naturally begin to stay down. If you ignore my advice in favor of being that arrogant prick who keeps his chin up as though he's trying to smell a taller man's asshole, don't expect me to come visit you in the hospital.

MOVEMENT

When your opponent attacks, movement is your best line of defense. Blocking can certainly be effective, but why risk possible injury when you can get out of the way? In addition to avoiding an unnecessary impact, evading an attack using movement is also an excellent way to disrupt your opponent's balance. If he expects to transfer his forward energy into a target, and then misses,

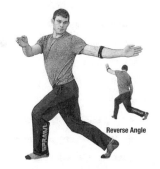

Reverse Angle

When fighting, never do this.

he'll often lose his footing, allowing you to quickly capitalize on his compromised positioning.

Movement is also essential to every attack. Without proper footwork, you'll never hit a damn thing. You don't want to be that douche bag who fires off elaborate combinations while standing ten feet away from his opponent. In addition to burning needless energy, it makes you look like a special-needs kid having a private battle with a gang of imaginary Mutant Ninja Turtles. Below, I offer some tips about footwork and movement that will make you harder to hit, your strikes more effective, and your takedowns a lot easier to manage.

spitting TIP #9: STANCE IN MOTION

When you move about the cage or ring, you always want to maintain your stance. If your feet get spread too far apart or you lean too far to one side or the other, your base and balance will be compromised. In addition to making you vulnerable to your opponent's attacks, it will also be difficult to execute attacks and counterattacks of your own. Although maintaining your stance while circling, advancing, and retreating can be difficult when you start out, there are ways to improve in this department. One such way is to tie a shoulder's-width length of rope between your legs while shadowboxing. After a few weeks of this, you'll be surprised at how much your footwork has improved.

get off my **TIP #10: NEVER CROSS YOUR FEET**

As a rule of thumb, you never want to cross your feet because it compromises your balance. To prevent this from happening, always begin by stepping the foot that is closest to the direction you want to head. For example, if you want to move to your right, step with your right foot first and then slide your left foot in the same direction to maintain your stance. The same rule applies when moving toward your left, forward, and backward. When you follow this simple rule, you will never have a problem crossing your feet.

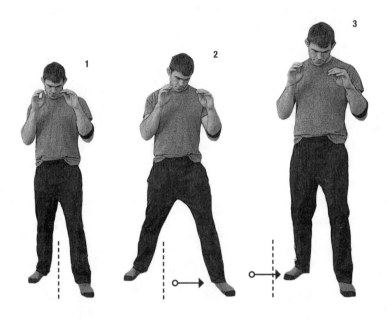

Wanting to move to my left, I step my left foot toward my left side. Once accomplished, I reestablish my fighting stance by sliding my right foot toward my left. If you look closely at the photos, you'll notice that moving in this manner actually makes you a larger person. Seriously. When I began fighting, I was five nine, like the coauthor of this book. Now I'm six eight. It's all in how you move… By the way, I was trying to set the world record for the number of different fonts used in a book, but my editor shut me down. However, I managed to sneak this one by him. Cool, isn't it? It's the font angry pirates use.

hidden TIP #11: CREATING ANGLES

Creating angles utilizing footwork is a very important aspect of fighting. When you are standing square with your opponent, it can be very difficult to land a strike or score a takedown because his lines of defense are directly in front of you. If you throw a punch to his face, he can block it with his arms. If you shoot in for a takedown, he can sprawl his hips straight back. Instead of confronting his defensive lines head-on, it's better to get around them. This can be accomplished by utilizing footwork to reposition your body off to his side. The goal is to create a brief moment where your hips are facing him but his hips are facing away from you. Before he can turn and once again square up with your body, you launch an attack from your new angle. The better you get at creating dominant angles, the more success you will have with your offensive techniques.

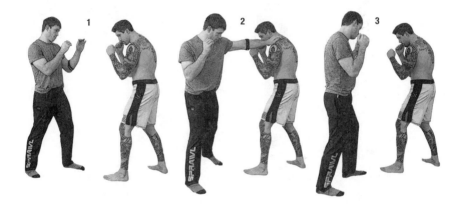

1) With my hips square with Neil's hips, it is difficult for me to break through his defenses.
2) As I throw a jab to distract Neil, I step my right foot toward the outside of his left foot.
3) I square my hips with Neil's left side by rotating my body in a counterclockwise direction. Before he can turn to face me, I will throw a strike or execute a takedown.

thick shaft, tiny **TIP #12: STANDARD VS. SOUTHPAW**

When you fight an opponent in an opposite stance, which means he has his opposite foot forward, the goal is to position your lead foot to the outside of his lead foot. For example, if he has his right foot forward and you have your left foot forward, you want to position your left foot to the outside of his right foot. Accomplishing this gives you a dominant angle from which to attack and allows you to score with a greater percentage of your strikes and takedowns.

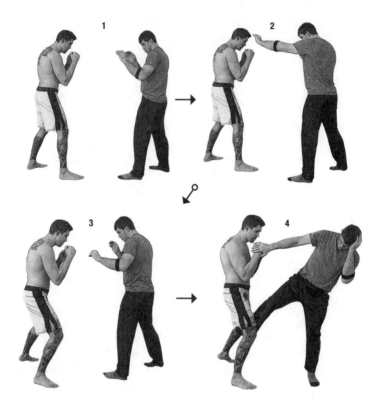

1) I'm in a traditional stance, and Neil is in a southpaw stance. 2) As I throw my left hand into Neil's face to blind him, I step my left foot to the outside of his right foot, giving me a dominant angle of attack. 3) Neil steps his right foot to the outside of my left foot to eliminate my dominant angle. 4) While Neil's weight is still on his right leg, I throw a right Thai kick to his inner right thigh. 5) Never ask Erich Krauss to Photoshop shit. Look at the first picture in the sequence above. Does that look like a foot? No, it does not. It looks like a talon of some sort. If you could do me a favor, e-mail Erich at authorerichkrauss@ hotmail.com and tell him what a retard he is. I'll owe you one. I mean, the guy found the time to remove the word sprawl from my pants, which cost me sponsorship money, but he was too busy to fix my foot? What kind of a guy does that?

mushroom TIP #13: SENSE OF DISTANCE

Having awesome strikes and blocks means nothing without a keen sense of distance. It's not an easy trait to develop, especially for guys who spend all their time striking the heavy bag. Don't get me wrong; working on the heavy bag can do wonders for your punches and kicks, but it does very little to prepare you for a live opponent who knows how to use his feet. To develop your sense of distance, you have to spend an ample amount of time sparring and drilling footwork with a training partner. One of the more helpful drills is to stand into the pocket with your opponent and track his movements. If he comes forward, you move backward. If he moves to his left, you follow him by moving to your right. At first, no strikes should be thrown. Your only goal is to remain in striking range by shadowing your opponent's movements. Once you get comfortable, add very light strikes into the mix. With time, you will automatically react to your opponent's movements, even when sparring at full speed. At every moment in the fight, you'll know whether you are in or out of striking range, allowing you to utilize techniques accordingly.

slowly rub my TIP #14: DON'T CIRCLE INTO THE POWER

When your opponent is standing with his left foot forward and his right foot back, he will be able to throw much more powerful strikes from his right side. His right cross will pack more power than his left jab, and his right kick will pack more power than his lead left kick. For this reason, you always want to avoid circling into your opponent's power side when in striking range. There are, of course, exceptions to this rule, but when first starting out, it's generally not a rule you want to break. It's okay to circle toward his power side as long as you create enough distance, but if your sense of distance is off, there is a very good chance that you'll eat a powerful shot. So to reiterate, if your opponent's right foot is back, circle toward his left side when in striking range, and if his left foot is back, circle toward his right when in striking range.

zipper caught my fucking **TIP #15: PRIMARY TARGETS**

The goal in any fight is to inflict the maximum amount of damage with every strike you throw. In order to accomplish this, you must first know what the optimal targets are. I've included a list below, but it is important to note that I've only included targets legal in MMA. If you're in a street fight, gouging your opponent's eyes and soccer-kicking his gonads are not just fair game, but highly encouraged.

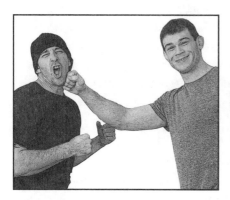 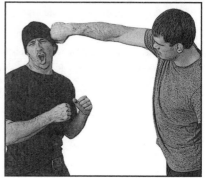

THE JAW

Striking your opponent square in the chin with your fist or shin can produce a devastating knockout. It causes the neck to jerk violently, which drives the brain against the skull and temporarily puts your opponent to sleep. When you strike the chin hard enough, sometimes it will cause your opponent's muscles to spasm, making his arms and legs shudder like a dying cockroach. Striking the chin in this fashion also sometimes causes your opponent to shit himself.

THE TEMPLE

It's possible to knock your opponent out cold by landing a hard strike to the temple, but most of the time it will cause a flash knockout, which a lot of people refer to as "seeing stars." The difference between a knockout and a flash knockout is that flash knockouts are easier to recover from, making it important that you continue to whale on your opponent until the referee or cops pull you off.

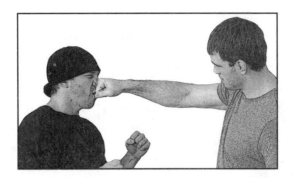

THE NOSE

Breaking your opponent's nose is awesome. It causes his eyes to water and blood to drain down the back of his throat, which impairs his breathing. Although it's not a fight finisher, it will usually steal a portion of his heart, cause him to fatigue faster, and disrupt his focus, which makes him vulnerable to other strikes. It also temporarily makes him uglier than you, which is good.

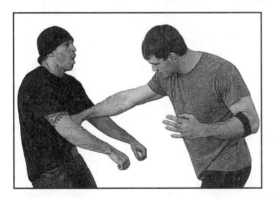

THE SOLAR PLEXUS

The solar plexus is located in the center of the sternum. When you strike this area of the body, it will usually steal your opponent's wind and cause him to drop his defenses. Sometimes you can even cause enough damage to get your opponent to quit, but this is rare.

LIVER AND KIDNEY

Striking these vital organs not only knocks the wind out of your opponent, but it also causes him an immediate burst of pain that will affect him long after the fight is over. To strike the region that contains the liver and kidney, target the soft tissue between your opponent's rib cage and hips on the sides of his body. The best strikes for the job are circular ones, such as Thai kicks and hooks.

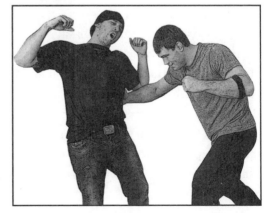

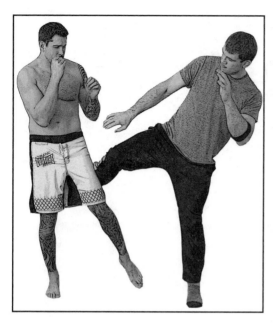

SCIATIC NERVE

The sciatic nerve runs down the side of the thigh, and the best weapon to damage it is a circular Thai kick. Although landing one kick to this sensitive area usually won't cause much damage, landing ten of them will. For the best results, you want to target the same area on your opponent's thigh over and over. As the fight progresses, your opponent will find it increasingly difficult and painful to put his weight on his leg. Not only does this limit his offensive movements, but it also draws his entire focus to the injured area, creating an opportunity to land other strikes, such as punches to his face.

TIP # 16: CONTACT POINTS

When people get into a fight, the majority of the time they will instinctively use their fists. This is primarily due to the control we have over our hands. We use them for just about everything—writing, driving, groping a massive set of titties, and, in your case, excessive masturbation. While your fists are certainly formidable weapons, they tend to shatter quite easily. I'm sure if you looked up the statistics, you'd find that the most common injury in MMA is broken hands. Punches are also quite easy for your opponent to spot because they are generally thrown from eye level. To avoid injury and become a more unpredictable scrapper, it is important to learn how to use the other weapons your body has come equipped with. However, you want to master each weapon before you attempt to use it in a fight. If you learn how to throw a Thai kick on Tuesday, you probably won't want to pull it out of your arsenal in a fight on Friday night. Just as it took you years to learn how to gain proper control over your hands, it can take years to learn how to throw effective kicks and knee and elbow strikes. Like everything in fighting, it just takes time. Below, I've included a list of your body's primary weapons that are legal in MMA. Once you've mastered these primary weapons, I suggest learning how to use your secondary weapons, such as the shoulder, which can be used in the clinch, and the palm, which can be used to deliver the highly touted pimp slap.

THE FIST

When throwing punches, always strike with the knuckles of your index and middle fingers. In addition to limiting the damage caused to your hand, it allows you to maximize the energy transference between your arm and your opponent's face . . . In short, it allows you to inflict more damage.

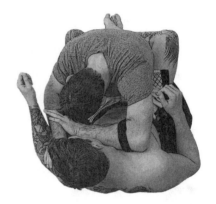

THE FOREARM

When you assume a top position on the ground, the forearm can be used as a grinding stone to crush and rearrange your hideous mug. In wrestling, this technique is commonly referred to as the cross-face.

TIP OF THE ELBOW

The tip of the elbow is responsible for opening more cuts than any other weapon. For the best results, throw your elbow along a downward, arching trajectory toward your opponent's face. If your goal is to draw blood, you want to graze your opponent's face with the tip of your elbow rather than land a solid blow.

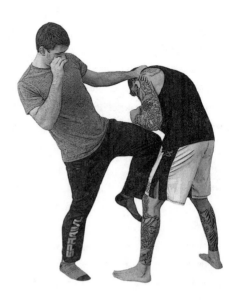

TIP OF THE KNEE

The knee is the battering ram of the human body. When used properly, it can cause severe damage to your opponent's legs, body, face, or cock 'n balls.

THE SHIN

When throwing kicks, you do not want to strike your target with your foot. You want to connect with your shin. Not only will this cause your opponent more damage, but it will also reduce the damage you suffer should your opponent check your kick. It's best to land with the inside portion of your shin where the bone is the thickest. If you land with the outside, you risk damaging the muscle tissue that runs down the side of your leg.

BALL OF FOOT

When you throw a straight front kick, you can strike your target using either the ball or heel of your foot. Striking with the ball allows you to cover more distance, but it won't produce as great an impact.

HEEL

The heel is used as a weapon when you throw front kicks, side kicks, back kicks, or stomp on a grounded opponent. To cause the most damage, flex your foot upward. This limits the surface area of your weapon and makes your heel as sharp as possible.

here, let me spit on my **TIP #17: SENSE OF TIMING**

"Sense of timing" is your ability to anticipate or predict your opponent's movements. It is referred to as a sense because it is not something you think about—it is more of a reaction. If your opponent moves, you do not think about that movement, you react to it either offensively or defensively. While sparring frequently will help your sense of timing for striking on your feet, it is also very important to develop this sense for ground fighting. Unless you have superhuman strength, you can't force techniques. To be effective, you have to use your opponent's movements and reactions to your movements to your advantage, and the only way you can accomplish this is with timing. I don't care if you only know a handful of techniques—if you have a good sense of timing, you'll submit your opponents more often than someone who knows every technique in the book but has awful timing. I'm not saying that you shouldn't focus on technique; all I'm saying is that you shouldn't ignore the importance of timing. To help improve in this area, you should spar and conduct timing drills on the ground as often as possible. (Note: Siblings, significant others, and spouses can make worthy sparring partners—chances are your little bro or lady friend have a few scores they'd like to settle, so you may not have to look too far for an opponent. Why go across the street when you can go across the hall? Or the bed . . .)

caress my **TIP #18 COMBINATIONS**

If your opponent is an experienced fighter, throwing single-strike attacks usually won't get you very far. In order to be effective, you have to string your strikes together to form fluid combinations. The goal is to make each strike set up the one to follow. For example, you throw a jab to your opponent's face to momentarily blind him and force him to raise his arms in defense. This sets you up to throw a powerful cross to his body. Upon impact, the cross knocks the air out of your opponent and causes him to bend forward, which in turn sets you up to throw a knee to his face. Landing the knee with power will discombobulate your opponent and knock him off balance, which allows you to finish the combination with a takedown. Unleashing a series of strikes like this is the best way to keep your opponent on the defensive. The same principle applies when fighting on the ground. If you latch onto your opponent's arm and try to apply a *kimura* submission, chances are he will defend against it. However, his defense makes him vulnerable to an armbar on the opposite side. If he defends against the armbar, you can immediately transition back to the *kimura*. But I get ahead of myself. Simply put, when you string submissions or strikes together, it's just a matter of time until you get one step ahead of your opponent.

I think you just kicked my **TIP #19 FEINTS (FOR THE VOCABULARILY CHALLENGED . . . THESE ARE "FAKES.")**

The goal of a feint is to trick your opponent into thinking you're attacking with a specific technique in order to generate a reaction. For example, you drop your elevation as though you are shooting in for a takedown, causing your opponent to drop his hands low to defend against your shot. However, instead of following through with the takedown, you quickly increase your elevation and capitalize on your opponent's unprotected head by throwing an overhand right. Another example is to throw a fake cross to get your opponent to react to that specific punch, and then quickly throw a lead hook. The goal is to commit enough to the feint to get your opponent to react to it, but not commit so much that it jeopardizes your follow-up attack.

under all that foreskin you'll find the TIP #20 LOW-HIGH PRINCIPLE

The low-high or high-low principle of attack is another excellent way to increase the effectiveness of your strikes. For example, you throw a kick aimed at your opponent's body to pull his focus downward, and then immediately follow up by throwing a punch aimed at his head. It works just as well the other way around—throw a punch at your opponent's head to pull his focus upward, and then follow up with a kick to his lower body. There are literally thousands of different low-high and high-low combinations that you can string together, and I strongly suggest finding the ones that work best for you. If you're like most fighters, you will find that it dramatically increases the percentage of strikes you land clean.

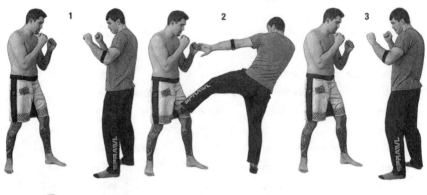

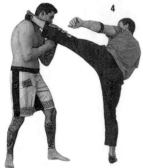

1) I'm squared off with Neil. 2) To draw his attention to the lower half of his body, I throw a left kick to the inside of his left leg.
3) I reestablish my fighting stance.
4) With Neil focusing on protecting his leg, I throw a left Thai kick to his head.

a leper fucks a hooker; in addition to giving her two hundred bucks, he also gave her a **TIP #21 KICKING A RETREATING OPPONENT**

Throwing kicks can be quite dangerous in MMA because you expose yourself to takedowns. For this reason, it's best to throw them when your opponent's balance is compromised or he's retreating. If you attempt to throw a kick to your opponent's body while he is stationary or moving forward, not only does he have the ability to knock you off balance by shooting in, but he can also catch your kick and haul you to the mat or land a powerful punch to your grille.

INCORRECT	CORRECT
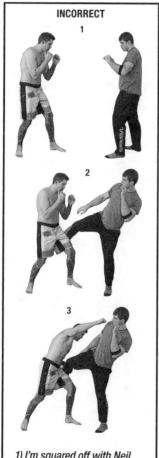	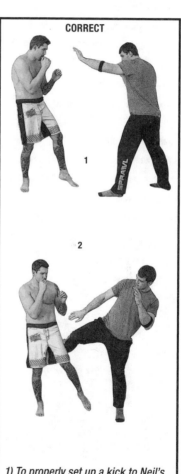
1) I'm squared off with Neil. 2) Neil advances, and I make the mistake of throwing a Thai kick to his lead leg. 3) With his body moving forward, he counters my kick by throwing an overhand right.	1) To properly set up a kick to Neil's lead leg, I throw a jab, forcing him to retreat. 2) I follow up with a Thai kick to Neil's lead leg. With his body moving backward, it is difficult for him to counter with a strike or takedown.

hidden TIP #22 TEMPO

Tempo or rhythm is often overlooked, but it is very important in fighting. Certain martial arts such as Muay Thai actually play music with a steadily increasing beat to create the tempo of a fight. Obviously this doesn't occur in MMA, but it doesn't mean rhythm is any less important. When you throw a combination, you want to create a tempo with your strikes. Once your opponent falls in turn with that tempo, suddenly breaking it can catch him off guard. For example, you may throw a jab-cross-hook, which is a three-beat combination, and then pause for a brief moment before throwing a low kick. With your opponent working on the steady beat of your attack, the pause throws him off and you have a greater chance of landing your strike. By mastering specific cadences, you can better set up your strikes and counter your opponent's strikes.

brown turtle TIP #23 BREAKING YOUR OPPONENT'S RHYTHM

Just as you create a rhythm with your strikes, so will your opponent. In order to prevent him from throwing strike after strike to the beat of his own drum, it is in your best interest to break his rhythm. For example, if your opponent plans on throwing a jab-cross combination, which consists of two beats, you can disrupt his rhythm by countering his jab with a jab of your own. Striking him while he's between beats not only prevents him from throwing the cross, but it also disrupts his rhythm and gives you a chance to begin beating *your* drum.

ANGLE 1   ANGLE 2

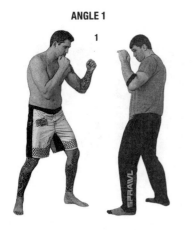
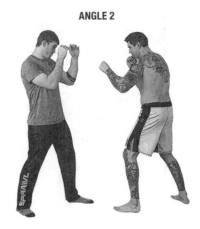

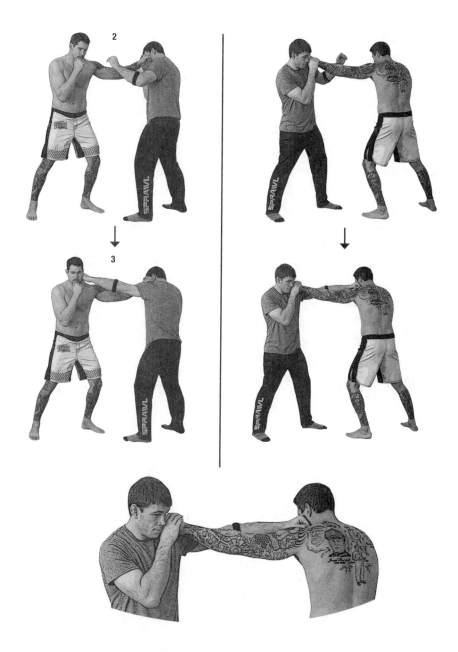

1) Neil and me are squared off in the pocket. 2) Neil throws a jab at my face. Instead of attempting a block, I evade his strike by shifting my weight toward my right side, dipping my head to my right, and parrying his fist to my left using my right hand. 3) As Neil's jab slips by the left side of my head, I throw a left jab. By striking him in the middle of my combination, I break his rhythm. To capitalize, I will immediately follow up with another strike.

TIP #24 ANSWER YOUR OPPONENT'S STRIKES

As I mentioned in the introduction to movement, you should always attempt to evade your opponent's strikes rather than block them. Although blocking oftentimes works, you absorb a good portion of the impact, risk your opponent's small glove wrapping around your blockade and striking your body and face, and make yourself vulnerable to his follow-up strikes. If you wrap your arms around your head and go into cover-up mode, it's only a matter of time until one of his punches connects solidly and puts you down. For this reason, don't ever let more than one strike go answered. If you block an opponent's punch, hit him before he can throw another.

TIP #25 BREATHING FOR STRIKING

When you strike, you always want to quickly exhale your air. In traditional arts, they call this something like "releasing your chi." I always thought releasing your chi was something else entirely, so I'm just going to call it smart. In addition to maximizing the power of your strike, it also prepares your body for counterstrikes. If your lungs are full of air and your opponent lands a strike to your chest, it can steal your wind and remove a large portion of your will to fight. To break the habit of holding your breath, every time you punch the mitts or kick the Thai pads, release a semiviolent shout that takes your air with it. You'll sound like one of those meatheads that try to get everyone in the gym to witness how much they can bench-press by grunting, but it will pay off when you step into the ring.

TIP #26 CLINCH-PUSH AND -PULL

When tied up in the clinch, you can always generate a reaction out of your opponent by either pushing into him or pulling him into you. If you push, almost a hundred percent of the time he will resist by pulling back, which allows you to release your pressure and immediately execute a forward throw or takedown. If you pull, he will almost always resist by pushing, which allows you to release your pressure and execute a backward throw or takedown. However, in order to effectively pull off either setup, you must develop an amazing sensitivity to your opponent's reactions. The instant he resists your push or pull, you must release your pressure and execute your offensive technique in the same direction as his resistance. If your timing is off, your opponent will be able to recover or launch an attack of his own.

MUAY THAI CLINCH

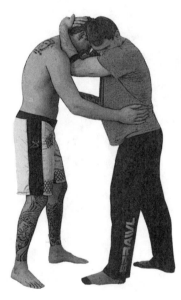

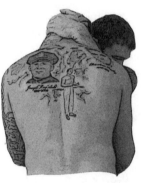

Moving into close range, I cup my right hand around the back of Neil's, and then cup my left hand over my right hand. To disrupt his balance, I pull his head down with my hands, and to prevent him from securing a body lock or shooting in for a takedown, I pinch my elbows together and drive them into his shoulders. From here, I can deliver power knees to his midsection.

TIP #27 GRECO, THAI, AND DIRTY BOXING

There are three primary clinching positions that are important for every mixed martial artist to learn—the Greco clinch, the Muay Thai clinch, and the dirty-boxing clinch. The Greco clinch focuses on upper-body control, which allows you to utilize attacks such as throws, body locks, and takedowns. The Muay Thai clinch focuses on head control, which allows you to off-balance your opponent and land brutal strikes with knees and elbows. The dirty-boxing clinch involves securing a collar tie with one hand to keep your opponent off balance while at the same time using your free hand to land repeated punches to his face and body. In order to be effective from the clinch, you must not only learn the basics of each of these clinching styles, but also learn how to blend them together in such a way that you can transition back and forth between them.

GRECO: DOUBLE UNDERHOOK BODY LOCK

CORRECT

INCORRECT

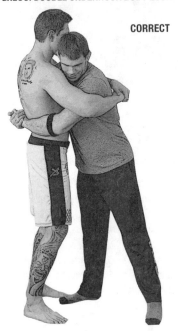 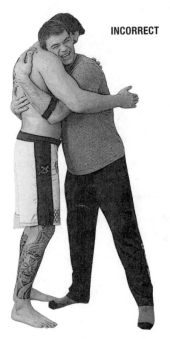

To secure a body lock, I dive my arms underneath Neil's arms, clasp my hands together in the small of his back, and then pull his hips into my body. From here, I can execute a number of effective takedowns.

This is not a body lock. This is man love at its finest. I know, very little difference. It's all in hand positioning. If your hands are clasped together, consider it a Greco-Roman clinch. If your hands are open, gently caressing your opponent's back, consider it extremely gay.

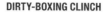

DIRTY-BOXING CLINCH

To establish the dirty-boxing clinch, I wrap one hand around the back of Neil's head and drive my elbow into his shoulder. To cause damage, I use my control to push and pull him off balance, circle around him, and repeatedly sock him in the face with my free hand.

TIP #28 INSIDE CONTROL

No matter which style of clinch you are playing—Greco, Thai, or dirty boxing—you always want to position your arms to the inside of your opponent's arms because it gives you dominant control. This is often a difficult chore. If your opponent is an experienced fighter, he, too, will attempt to secure inside control. Whoever wins this battle will be able to cause more damage with his strikes and execute more effective takedowns. There are many ways to secure inside control, such as obtaining double collar ties, double underhooks, or inside biceps ties. In addition to knowing how to secure each position, you must also learn how to escape each position should your opponent get the upper hand.

TIP #29 ALWAYS ON YOUR SIDE

You never want to lie flat on your back because it allows your opponent to control your body and punish you with strikes. By turning onto your side, you create space, and that space allows you to move and create openings to escape.

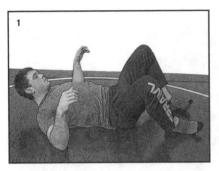

I'm lying flat on my back, which seriously hinders my mobility. If my opponent can keep me pinned in this position, he'll have a greater chance of landing effective strikes and locking in submissions.

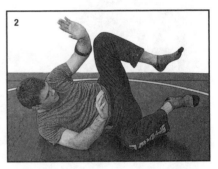

To increase my offensive and defensive options, I turn onto my right side.

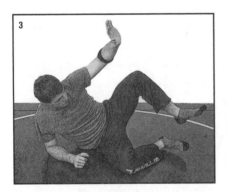

I come up onto my right elbow, increasing my mobility even more.

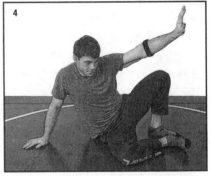

I post my right hand on the mat. From this position, I can escape back to my feet, execute an assortment of sweeps, or transition to a more dominant position.

TIP #30 SUBMISSION, SWEEP, OR GET UP

When you're stuck on your back with an opponent between your legs in your guard, you should have three things on your mind—submission, sweep, or get the fuck up. If you lie there thinking about how you forgot to feed your dog, you're pretty much locking yourself into an ass kicking. You have to remember that mixed martial arts is not a grappling match—your opponent can beat the living hell out of you. This should give you a sense of urgency and force you to move until you accomplish one of your three goals. Over the coming pages, I demonstrate several submissions, a couple of transitions, and a technique that you can use to escape back to your feet.

KIMURA SUBMISSION

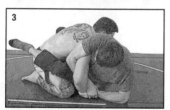

To prevent Neil from posturing up in my guard, I wrap my right hand around the back of his head and grab his right arm with my left hand.

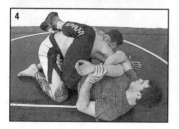

As Neil attempts to break my head and arm control and posture up, I slide my left hand down to his right wrist, plant my right foot on the mat, turn onto my left side, and reach my right arm over his left arm.

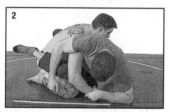

Maintaining a firm grip on Neil's right wrist using my left hand, I dive my right arm under his right arm and grab my left wrist with my right hand, establishing a figure-four grip.

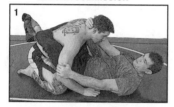

Scooting my hips toward my left side, I drop to my right shoulder, pull down on Neil's right arm using my right arm, and drive his right wrist up using my left hand. To prevent him from passing my guard, I have once again hooked my feet together. With a tremendous amount of pressure being applied to his right shoulder, he has no choice but to tap. Obviously if you successfully execute this in a no-holds-barred street fight, "tap" actually translates into your opponent screaming, "YOU'RE GONNA BREAK MY ARM!!! SWEET JESUS, YOU'RE GONNA BREAK MY FUCKIN' ARM!!! I WEAR SKIRTS <SOBBING> I . . . WEAR . . . SKIRTS <MORE SOBBING>."

OMAPLATA SUBMISSION

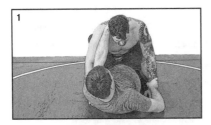

I have Neil in my closed guard. In an attempt to break my head and arm control and posture up, he places his hands on the mat and pushes off.

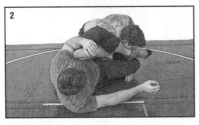

I turn onto my right side, scoot my hips toward my left side, throw my left leg over the back of Neil's right arm, and position my foot in front of his face. Notice how I have my left arm pinned to his right arm to prevent him from pulling it free.

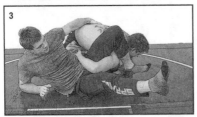

I pull my right leg out front underneath Neil's body, rotate my body ninety degrees, and wrap my left arm over his back to prevent him from escaping the submission by executing a forward roll.

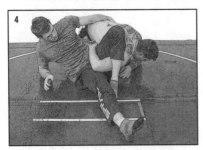

I wrap my leg tightly over Neil's right arm and begin sitting up.

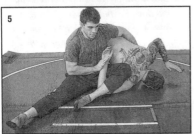

Sitting all the way up, I pin Neil's right shoulder to the mat by applying downward pressure with my right leg. To lock in the submission, I grab his right wrist with my right hand and drive it forward toward the mat. Do this right, and I hope the submitted has a willing love partner, because unless he's left-handed, masturbation will seem like climbing Everest in a blizzard.

OMAPLATA TRANSITION TO BACK

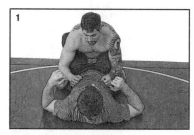

I have Neil in my closed guard.

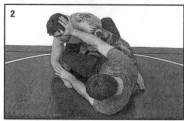

Turning onto my left side, I place my right foot on the mat, scoot my hips toward my right side, and drive my right hand into the left side of Neil's head to disrupt his balance.

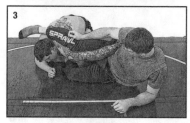

I attempt an omaplata submission by throwing my right leg over Neil's left arm, but he defends against the submission by pulling his arm free.

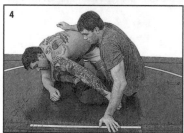

Instead of returning to the guard position, I use Neil's compromised positioning to post my left hand on the mat and reach my right arm over his back.

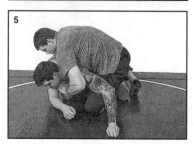

Before Neil has a chance to reestablish his base and balance, I come up onto my left knee and secure a body lock by wrapping my left arm over his left shoulder and under his body, wrapping my right arm around his right side, and clasping my hands together. From this position, I have numerous offensive options.

UNDERHOOK GET UP TO BACK

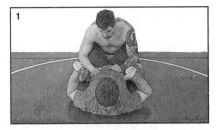

I have Neil in my closed guard.

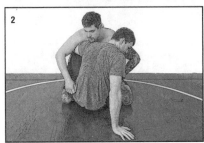

As Neil postures up to strike, I post my right hand on the mat, sit up with him, and dive my left arm underneath his right arm, securing an underhook.

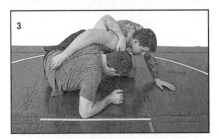

As I drop down to my right elbow, I turn onto my right side, scoot my hips toward my left, and drive my left arm downward into Neil's right arm, forcing him to lose balance and plant his left hand on the mat.

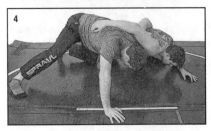

Posting my right hand and right foot on the mat, I come up onto my left knee and wrap my left arm over Neil's back.

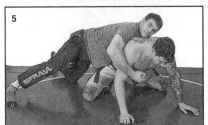

I slide my body and head out from underneath Neil's right arm, reposition my body over his back, and secure a body lock by clasping my hands together.

GET UP

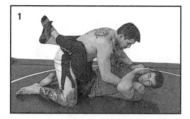

Neil is in my closed guard.

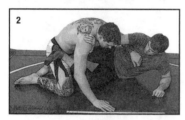

To create space, I place my right hand on Neil's right shoulder and drive him away from me. At the same time I turn onto my left side, post my left elbow on the mat, and move my left foot toward the front of his right hip.

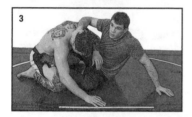

Planting my left foot on Neil's right hip to maintain space, I place my right hand on the back of his neck and post my left hand and right foot on the mat.

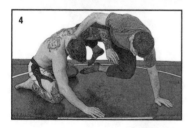

Pushing off the mat with my right foot, I drive my right hand down into the back of Neil's head, support my weight on my left hand, and leap my body out from underneath him.

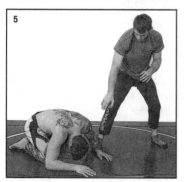

I plant my feet on the mat. From here, I will either back away or launch an attack. If this is a street fight, your decision will determine whether you're a martial artist or a fighter—I ain't judging.

TIP #31 POSTURE CONTROL

When your opponent postures up in your guard, he creates space between your body and his body. This is not good because it gives him the distance he needs to throw powerful strikes or work on transitioning to a more dominant position. To limit your opponent's offensive options, every time he sits up you want to immediately eliminate the space he created. This can be accomplished one of two ways—break him back down into your guard or sit up with him.

FULL GUARD TO BUTTERFLY GUARD

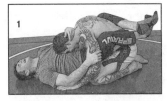

Neil is in my closed guard and I've secured head and arm control to keep him from posturing up.

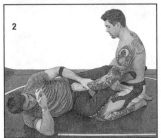

Neil breaks my head and arm control and postures up. To hinder him from throwing downward strikes, I immediately turn onto my right side, slide my left knee across his stomach, plant my right foot on his left hip, and grab his left arm with my left hand.

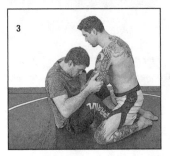

Using my left grip on Neil's left wrist, I sit up into him, grab the back of his left triceps with my right hand, and slide my feet between his legs to secure the butterfly guard.

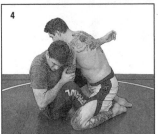

Maintaining my right grip on Neil's left triceps, I dive my left arm underneath his right arm to secure an underhook. Securing the butterfly guard in this fashion has given me all sorts of sweep options (i.e., ways to put the motherfucker on his back).

TIP #32 REAR NAKED CHOKE

Chokes are the most dangerous submissions because rather than threatening your joints, they threaten blood flow to your brain, which can result in death, shitting yourself, or both. To protect your neck, always keep your chin pinned to your chest. If at any point your opponent should obtain a dominant position and apply a choke, immediately latch onto his choking arm with both hands and rip it away from your neck. Do not make the mistake of trying to escape the position before blocking the choke because it only takes a few seconds to pass out. Once you have removed your opponent's arm from your neck, that's when you focus on improving your position. If the roles are reversed and you are in a position to choke your opponent, immediately go for the finish (sweep the leg, Johnny). If your opponent's defenses are extremely sharp, instead of wasting energy trying to lock it in, move on to strikes or another submission. As soon as you have your opponent distracted, return to the choke.

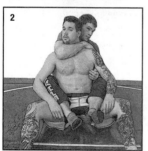

I've taken Neil's back and secured over-under control. If you should find yourself in Neil's shoes, you should immediately protect your neck by grabbing your opponent's choking arm with both hands and pulling it downward.

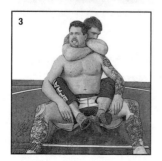

Neil fails to protect his neck, so I immediately begin transitioning to the rear naked choke by cupping my right hand behind his left shoulder to secure my arm in place and pulling my left arm out from underneath his left arm. Although it looks like I'm pinching his nipple in this photo, this is not a part of the technique. If you attempt this, it will either anger your opponent or lead to heavy moaning.

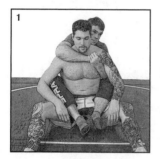

To secure the rear naked choke, I grab my left bicep with my right hand and cup my left hand around the back of Neil's head. To cut off the blood flow to his brain, I drive his head downward using my left hand and squeeze my arms tight.

TIP #33 NEVER LET YOUR LIMBS STRAY

Always keep your limbs drawn tight to your body. If you get into the bad habit of reaching for your opponent or straightening your limbs, you give him an open invitation to transition to an armbar or leg lock.

ARMBAR FROM MOUNT

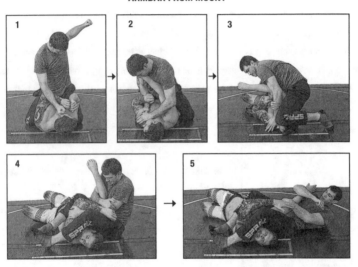

1) I've secured the mount position on Neil and begin striking him repeatedly in the face. 2) Neil breaks a cardinal rule by extending his right arm into my body in an attempt to push me off of him. 3) The instant Neil extends his right arm, I wrap my right arm over his right arm and then grab my left forearm with my right hand, securing his arm to my body. At the same time I post my right foot on the mat, rotate my body in a clockwise direction, and drive my left knee across his face. 4) I step my left foot to the left side of Neil's head and drop down to my butt. Notice how I have slid my right hand up to my left biceps to keep his arm pinned to my chest. 5) As I drop to my back, I straighten Neil's right arm by sliding the crook of my right arm up to his wrist. To finish the armbar, I pull his right arm toward my chest, drive my legs into his face and body to keep them pinned to the mat, and elevate my hips. Tap, tap, TAP!

TIP #34 BODY-BODY-HEAD

When you're on top in your opponent's guard, always put together combinations that create openings for power shots. A perfect example of this is the body-body-head combination. The majority of the time, your opponent will have his arms elevated to protect his head, allowing you to throw hard punches at his unprotected ribs. After absorbing a few blows, he will most likely drop his elbow to protect his ribs. The instant he drops his arm, you have a perfect opportunity to throw a hard strike to his unprotected head.

TIP #35 PASSING THE GUARD

When you're in your opponent's guard, never lie on top of him and stall. Chances are you worked hard to secure a takedown and reach this position, and stalling will accomplish nothing more than forcing the referee to stand you back up. To prevent such an outcome, distract your opponent with strikes and work on passing his guard to a more dominant position such as side control or mount. When you are successful, you not only score points on the judges' scorecards, but you also attain a position that makes it much easier to lock in submissions or cause damage with strikes.

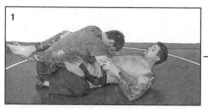

I'm in Neil's closed guard. Instead of remaining in this position, I'm going to pass to side control.

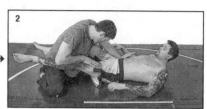

To create space, I dig my left knee into the center of Neil's buttocks, drive my left hand down into his abdomen, and lean back. As my actions force his legs apart, I begin pressing down on his left leg with my right hand (if he giggles or moans in ecstasy, flick him in the nads).

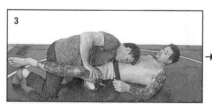

I drop my body on top of Neil and force his left leg toward the mat using my right hand.

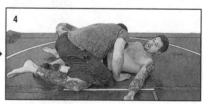

I slide my right knee over Neil's left leg.

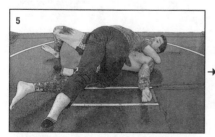

Keeping Neil's left leg pinned to the mat using my right leg, I wrap my right arm around the back of his head and step my left leg over his right leg.

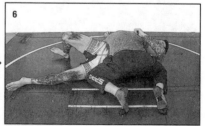

Having passed Neil's guard, I slide my right knee underneath his left shoulder and pin my left knee against his left hip. From this position, I have a greater opportunity to land strikes, lock in a submission, or transition to an even more dominant position.

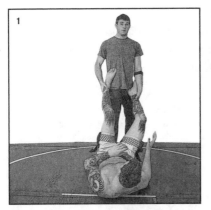

PASSING THE DOWNED GUARD

There are many ways to end up standing in front of a downed opponent. You can stand up in his guard, execute a throw or take-down, or your opponent could simply fall to his back in an attempt to bait you down into his guard. If your goal is to keep the fight standing, backing away from your opponent will usually cause the referee to stand him back up. But if you want to engage him in the ground game, it's in your best interest to pass his guard. In this situation, I set up the pass by grabbing his feet with my hands.

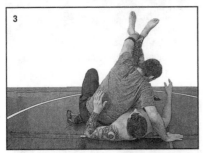

Quickly rotating my body in a counterclockwise direction, I cross Neil's left leg over the top of his right and move his feet toward my left side.

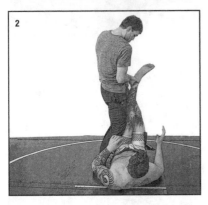

Maintaining control of Neil's right leg using my left hand, I drop down to my right hip and place my right hand to the right of his head.

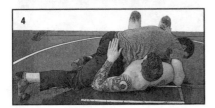

Having cleared Neil's legs, I drop my weight down on him to prevent him from scrambling, move my left arm to the right side of his body, and pin my left knee to his left hip.

TIP #36 STAY POSTURED

When in your opponent's guard, always remain postured. Not only will this make it more difficult for him to catch you in a submission, but it also allows you to generate a shitload of power with your strikes.

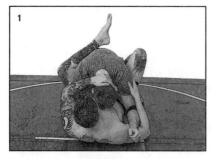

I've broken down in Neil's guard. To improve my effectiveness with strikes, I need to posture up.

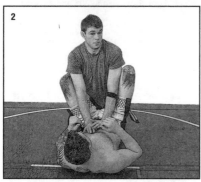

I dig my palms into Neil's abdomen and posture up by straightening my arms.

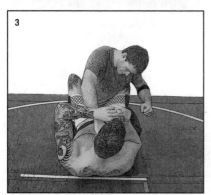

Having postured up, I rotate my body in a counterclockwise direction and throw a powerful right to Neil's face.

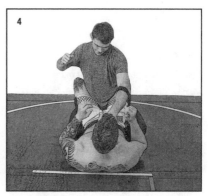

Immediately after landing the cross, I rotate my body in a clockwise direction and throw a powerful left to Neil's face.

TIP #37 FOLLOW THE HIPS

When you're on top in your opponent's guard, he will constantly shift his hips from side to side to create space. If you allow him to create that space, his chances of sweeping you to your back or locking in a submission improve greatly. To hinder his goal, eliminate all space he creates by tracking the movement of his hips. When done properly, your opponent's chances of successfully executing a sweep or submission drop dramatically.

TIP #38 LOW-RISK VS. HIGH-RISK TECHNIQUES

Low-risk techniques are generally simple techniques. With just a few steps involved, your opponent will have less time to defend against them. High-risk techniques are generally complex and flashy, and if you attempt one and fail, it will often leave you in a compromising position. For this reason, the majority of techniques you execute in the cage should be simple and low risk. However, if your opponent is broken mentally and physically, and your goal is to earn the submission or knockout of the night (which could get you both a bonus and an open invitation to fight another day—winning by decision don't guarantee nothin'), flashy techniques can come in handy. But you must always ask yourself if the juice is worth the squeeze.

TIP #39 STAY RELAXED

Whether you are striking or grappling, always stay relaxed. When you're tight, your attacks are slower, you tire quickly, and your reactions are delayed.

TIP #40 RECOVERY BREATHING

When tired or fatigued, take deep breaths in through your nose and exhale out your mouth. It also helps to take air in using your stomach rather than your chest because it allows you to absorb more oxygen. If you take choppy breaths, it will take twice as long to recover.

TIP #41 DIET

Just like you wouldn't put shit in the gas tank of your car, don't put shit into your body. If you want to perform at your best, put high-octane fuel into your system. (Yes, that analogy was very, very lame.) Knowing what foods to base your diet on doesn't take a brain surgeon—clean meats and loads of fruits and vegetables. However, I do not follow this in the least. I can get away with this because I have different genetics than you. My body works best when fueled by cookies, ice cream, and blue cotton candy. I'm like an elf.

TIP #42 THE GOLDEN RULE

Remember, anything that works is valid. If someone tells you that a technique sucks ass, but it works for you, keep it in your arsenal. The goal is not to be like everyone else. The goal is to develop your own fighting style.

BOOK 6

THE VAULT OF SUPERSECRET TECHNIQUES

FUCK START THE HEAD

When I was on the *Fox and Friends* morning show a while ago, they wanted me to show them a fighting technique. I could have broken down an armbar or a rear naked choke, but that would have been lame. Wanting to leave a good impression, I showed them the technique demonstrated below. It's called Fuck Start the Head, and it's the proper way to break someone's neck. If you've watched any Steven Seagal movie, you probably think all you have to do is grab your attacker's chin in one hand, the back of his head in the other, and then end his life with a quick twist. That is complete horseshit and will never work. I mean, come on, Steven Seagal runs like a little girl, what makes you think he knows anything about breaking necks? If you buy into that shit, the only thing you'll ever break is your dick on another man's ass. So if you want to learn the proper way to snap a neck, learn Fuck Start the Head. It can be difficult to pull off on skilled athletes, but it works great against drunk assholes, really old people (frail bones), and wrestlers who shoot in with their hands down and their neck exposed.

TOTALLY INCORRECT

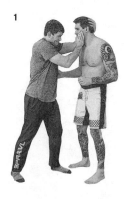
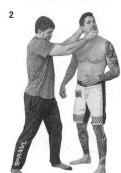
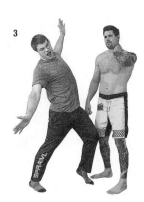

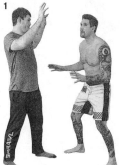

CORRECT

Blindly reaching out for your opponent's head is a good way to get punched in the face, so I prefer to set up the technique using a tactic called "twinkle fingers." All it takes is elevating your arms and moving your fingers in an excited fashion. This will draw your opponent's focus every single time, allowing you to go in for the kill.

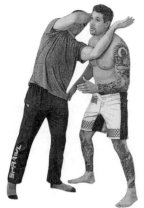

2

I slide my right arm across the right side of Neil's face. At the same time I slide my left forearm across the left side of his neck.

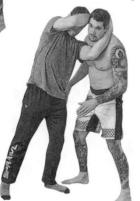

3

I cup the back of Neil's head with my left hand, and then wrap my right hand over the top of my left.

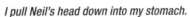

I pull Neil's head down into my stomach.

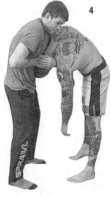

4

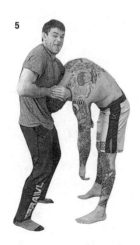

5

Thrusting my hips forward, I jerk my arms upward. With Neil's head pinned against my stomach, his neck experiences an upward torque that causes it to break. Just as anytime you kill someone, you must stick out your tongue to impress any chicks who happen to be standing around watching.

HOW TO FEND OFF A DOG ATTACK

As you can clearly tell from the photos below, dogs are vicious creatures that will tear your throat out just for shits and giggles. If you should have a head-to-head confrontation with one of these ruthless killing machines, do not attempt to apply the rear naked choke demonstrated earlier in the book. Dogs have very small heads because they are stupid, and if they manage to wiggle free of your hold, they will most likely latch onto your arm. A much safer approach is to reach an arm underneath the dog's body, cup your hand behind the jaw and around the neck, and apply pressure.

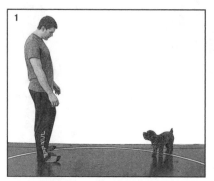

What's up, you little hairy bitch? You want a piece of Forrest, bitch! Huh, what'd you say? Talking shit? You want a piece of the Griff? You messing with the 702, sucka. (Yes, I talk about myself in the third person, and yes, I have given myself nicknames . . . You want a piece of the Griffendor, too?!?)

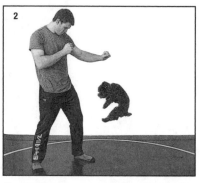

You don't scare me, white boy. I punk-slap ticks larger than you! I fuck guys like you at the pound. I'm coming, corn bread, I'm coming!

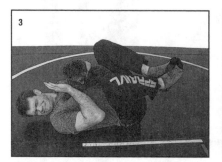

Ohhh, shit dog, get off me! Your breath. Oh God, your breath is like hot, fiery fire. You been eating cat shit or your own ass. It smells like a mixture of both. Uncle . . . I said uncle . . .

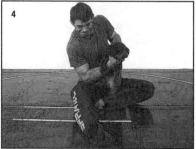

You cheater! You cried uncle and then went for my neck . . . Let me go! . . . Oooowww. I just shit on you . . . Fading . . . fading. Tell Sparkles I love her . . . Before I go, let me tell you the meaning of life . . . It's . . . it's . . . uurrggg.

THE GOOD OL' KNEE TO THE NUT SAC

When you walk up to some random guy on the street, it's quite easy to kick him in his junk because he's totally unsuspecting. However, when you're in a fight on the street or in the cage, usually your opponent will focus on protecting his happy place. If you throw a knee to the cock 'n balls, his legs will instinctively cross, preventing any damage. Utilizing the technique shown below will ensure contact, causing your opponent to drop to his knees and vomit for approximately half an hour (so, ladies, listen up). I know this technique works because I've seen Check Congo use it on a regular basis in the Octagon.

1

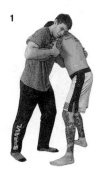

I'm tied up with Neil in the over-under clinch. It's a neutral position because we both have an overhook and an underhook. Instead of trying to pummel for a second underhook so I can secure a body lock, which is what honest fighters do, I plan to knee him as hard as I can in the satchel.

2

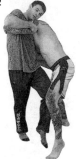

To set up the knee strike to the groin, I elevate Neil's left arm using my right hand, twist his body in a counterclockwise direction using my underhook, and strike his inner left thigh with my left knee. Not only do these actions throw him off balance, but they also spread his legs apart, clearing a pathway to his nuts.

3

With Neil's balance disrupted, I plant my left foot in front of me and slide my right foot back. If you're in a professional fight, this is the moment when you want to briefly glance around the cage to make sure the referee doesn't have a good visual of your opponent's package.

4

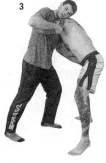

Before Neil can reacquire his balance and slide his legs together, I rocket my right knee forward into his twig and berries.

HOW TO FEND OFF A SWORD ATTACK

First off, never bring a knife to a sword fight. That's just plain stupid. A much better way to fight a guy with a sword is with your hands. In the sequence below, I demonstrate a hand-to-sword technique that Peruvian monks used to use for disarming Pirates. The reason I capitalized the word *pirate* is that they deserve respect for attacking Peruvian monks with just a sword during medieval times. At the very least, they should have used a machine gun. Anyway, the technique is supersecret, so if you talk your big brother into practicing it with you using your uncle's machete, do not tell your mother that you learned the technique from me. That would break the supersecret code and give you herpes for life.

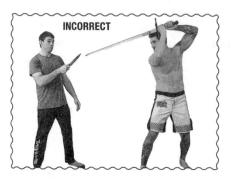

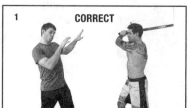

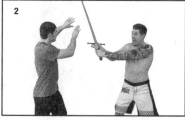

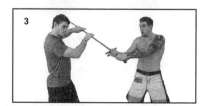

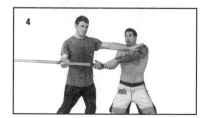

1) My attacker draws back his sword and swings it at me with all his might. Keeping my feet spread a shoulder's width apart, I open my hands in the direction of the blade. 2) I turn my face toward the advancing blade and slightly extend my arms. 3) I catch the hard steel in the web of my hands, thwarting the deadly strike. 4) Holding the sharp blade as tight as possible in my right hand, I render my opponent unconscious by delivering a savage knife strike to his throat. Next, I stab him with his own sword and begin plundering his small village on the icy, windswept shores of Scandinavia.

THE EYE GOUGE (FOR THE STREET ONLY)

Eye gouging should not be done with an open hand. In addition to telling everyone watching that you're a cheater, you also risk breaking your fingers. The proper approach is to extend your thumb slightly beyond a closed fist and punch your opponent in the center of his face. In addition to causing damage with your strike, your fist will usually slide off the bridge of your opponent's nose and allow your thumb to dig deep into his eye socket. Once you have him blinded, you immediately want to follow up with the Good Ol' Knee to the Nut Sac technique demonstrated earlier. (If you utilize this technique in the cage, you're not only a cheater, you're also a dirty piece of shit who deserves to die. When fighting for sport, never fuck with a man's eyes. That shit ends careers and will garner you an ample amount of haters, including me, for the rest of your life.)

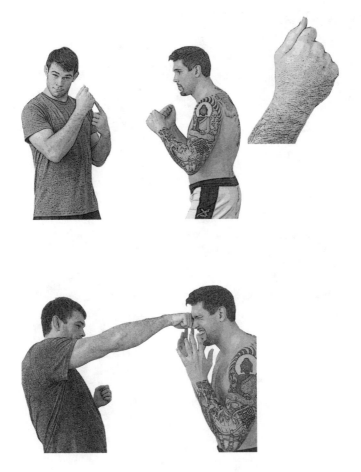

THE HOCKEY BEAT-DOWN

The Hockey Beat-down is basically the street version of the dirty-boxing clinch. Instead of hooking one hand around the back of your opponent's head, you latch onto the collar of his shirt or jacket. The trick to being effective with the technique is using your grip to constantly keep your opponent off balance. You want to push into him, throw a couple of strikes, pull him into you, throw a couple of strikes, circle and pull him with you, throw a couple of strikes. You get the point. What you don't want to do is grab your opponent's collar and then just stand there trying to punch him. With one of your hands tied up with your grip, he will be able to land some pretty solid blows to your face.

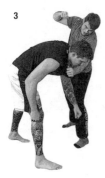

1   *I latch onto Neil's right collar, drive his shoulder back to disrupt his balance, and throw a right cross at his face.*

2

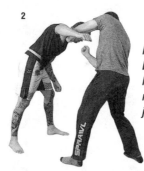

Keeping Neil off balance by pulling him forward, I land a right uppercut to his jaw.

3

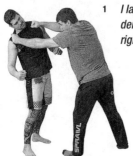

I circle to my right and pull Neil with me, further disrupting his base and balance. I use the opportunity to draw my right hand back.

4

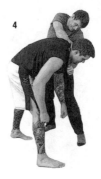

I land a savage right to Neil's left ear.
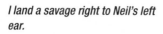

NO, *YOU* SHUT THE FUCK UP

This is an excellent technique to utilize when in a heated argument with your landlord or boss. By pointing a finger at your aggressor's face, you're pretty much assuring that he will point his finger back at you. The instant he does, latch onto that sucker and break it in half. It is important to note, however, that if you are in a serious fight, breaking your opponent's finger will most likely just piss him off. To prevent him from retaliating, kick him in the nuts while he is down on one knee.

1

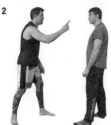

I point my finger into Neil's face to make him irate. To ensure that I get the reaction I desire, I add, "You're a greasy punk bitch, and I order you to be quiet."

2

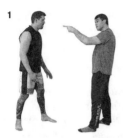

Neil takes the bait and points his finger back at me. He utters something about respect and how he's not afraid of me, but I'm not listening.

3

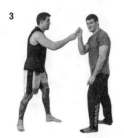

I grab Neil's finger with my right hand.

4

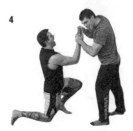

As I grab Neil's right wrist with my left hand, I break his finger with my right. To rub salt into the wound, I mutter, "How you like that, greasy punk bitch?!?!" Next, I will soccer-kick him in the groin.

ACQUIRING THE HEADLOCK

This is an excellent technique for putting your opponent into a headlock, which allows you to pulverize his face until it becomes unrecognizable. If you look at the photos in the sequence below, you'll notice that my hips are turned away from my opponent. This is to prevent him from grabbing my balls and applying severe downward pressure. Do not overlook technical detail. This technique works especially well on annoying children.

1

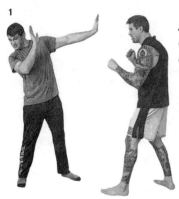

Angered, Neil approaches me with fists clenched. I outstretch my right hand, cover my face with my left hand, and turn my head away as though I'm cowering.

2

Lunging forward off my back foot, I wrap my left arm around Neil's head. Notice how my right hand is shielding the left side of my face.

3

I grab my shirt with my left hand, tightly securing Neil's head. Immediately I bend over, tug Neil off balance, and draw back my right fist.

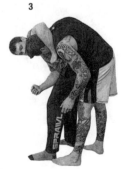

4

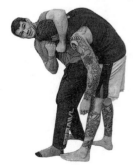

I land the first strike of many to Neil's face.

ESCAPING THE HEADLOCK

This is the most violent way to escape a headlock and it should be taught to every child at the age of five. It requires you to grab your opponent's package, which is unpleasant, but it is better than having your face repeatedly punched. FYI, this technique doesn't work when your aggressor is a woman.

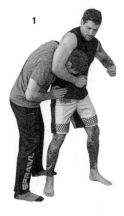

I've been captured in a headlock.

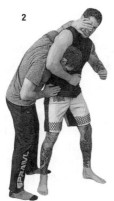

I reach my left arm over Neil's right shoulder and plant my hand on his face. For the best results, dig your fingers into your opponent's eyes.

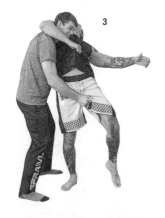

Forcing Neil's head backward using my left hand, I grab his nuts with my right hand and violently lift.

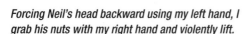

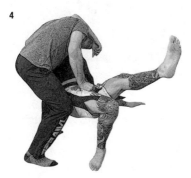

Still forcing Neil's head backward using my left hand, I yank upward on his nuts and lift his feet off the ground. The instant he hits the floor, he will curl into the fetal position and begin sobbing horribly. And I'll have a handful of nuts.

INSIDE TRIP

The Inside Trip is one of my favorite takedowns from the clinch, especially from the over-under position. The nice part about this technique is that it is relatively safe. There is little risk of getting kneed in the face because you don't have to drop your elevation, and if you fail, you can quickly recover and transition into another takedown.

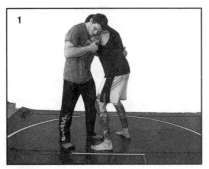

I'm tied up with Neil in the over-under clinch. With both Neil and me having an overhook and an underhook, this is a neutral position.

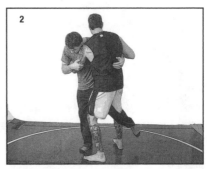

Rotating in a clockwise direction, I force Neil's weight off of his right leg by pulling on his left arm using my right hand and pushing into his body using my left arm. Once accomplished, I hook my left leg around the back of his right leg.

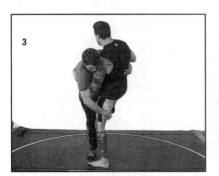

Throwing my left leg behind me, I reach down and grab the back of Neil's left leg with my right hand. As my left leg gets higher, Neil loses his balance and falls backward.

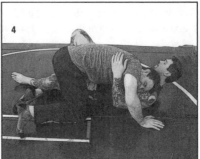

Neil falls to his back and I come down on top of him, landing in his half guard. The following photos, had we decided to put them in this book, thus making it a page longer (and thus WAY too long), depicted me posturing and delivering many punishing blows to Neil's head. I got a little carried away.

KNEE TO ELBOW

This is a very simple technique that you can use in the street or the cage. I tried to think up more shit to say about it, but as you probably realized by now, I'm not into padding my book with a bunch of fluff.

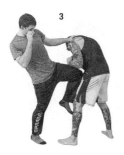

I'm squared off with Neil in my fighting stance.

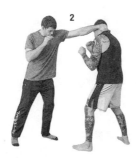

I shoot my left hand forward like I'm throwing a jab, but instead of socking Neil in the face, I wrap my hand around the back of his neck.

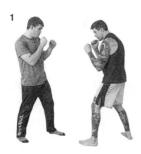

Pulling Neil's head toward me using my left hand, I drive my left knee into his midsection.

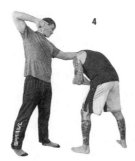

With Neil bent over from the knee strike, I draw my right elbow back.

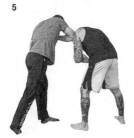

Rotating my hips in a counterclockwise direction, I land a downward elbow to the side of Neil's face.

COUNTERING STRIKES TO TAKEDOWN

A lot of fighters are in the habit of mirroring their opponent's strikes. For example, if you throw a Thai kick to your opponent's leg, there is a good chance he'll immediately throw a Thai kick to your leg. It's a subconscious way of saying, "Fuck you, bitch, I ain't letting you get one up on me." If I'm in a fight and I notice my opponent mirroring my attacks, I'll often use this to my advantage. Takedowns are a lot easier to execute successfully when your opponent throws punches because it hinders his ability to sprawl or counter with a knee to the face. So I'll throw a one-two punching combination, and the instant my opponent throws a one-two punching combination back, I'll drop underneath his punches and shoot in for a double leg takedown. It is important to notice that once I have my opponent's legs, I don't drive him straight back because it would place me in his guard. Instead, I drive him to the mat laterally, landing me in side control.

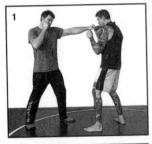

I throw a jab at Neil's chin.

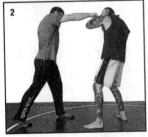

I throw a right cross.

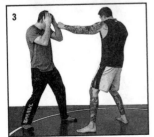

Having just eaten a one-two punching combination, Neil quickly fires off a jab.

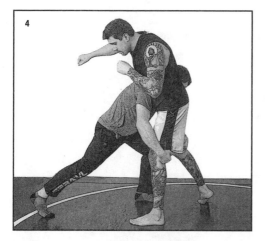

As Neil throws a right cross, I drop my elevation and shoot in underneath his punch, seizing the backs of his legs with my hands.

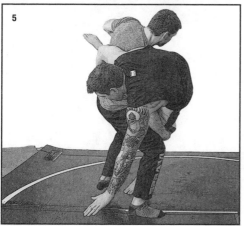

Instead of plowing Neil forward, I drive him to my right side by lifting his right leg off the mat with my left arm and trapping his left leg with my right arm.

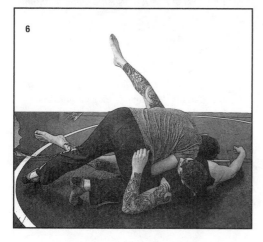

As Neil falls to his back, I come down with him and land in side control.

THE ASIAN DART

In today's MMA, a lot of opponents have very tight defense, especially when you take their back. To prevent you from establishing your hooks and flattening them bellydown on the mat, they'll keep their elbows pinned to their knees. And to keep you from locking in a rear naked choke, they'll keep their chin tucked to their chest. Although finding yourself up against such an opponent can be extremely frustrating, I have just the technique to remedy the situation. Now I have to warn you, it requires you to stick your thumb up your opponent's arse. Wrestlers call it "Checking the Oil," porn stars call it "The Thumb Blast." I call it the "Asian Dart" because I like to be different. No matter what you call it, the goal is the same—startle your opponent so severely that he raises his chin and allows you to lock in the choke.

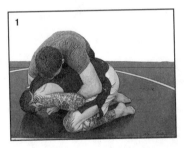

I'm extremely frustrated. I've claimed Neil's back, but he is balled up so tight I can't do shit. I can't secure my hooks, and I can't lock in a choke. Extreme times call for extreme measures, so I decide to employ the infamous Asian Dart.

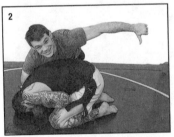

Keeping my weight on Neil's back to maintain control, I extend my left arm and point my thumb downward.

I drive my left thumb into Neil's ass, causing him to abandon his defensive tactics, elevate his head, and cry out in pain.

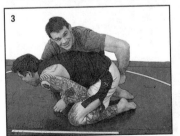

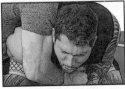

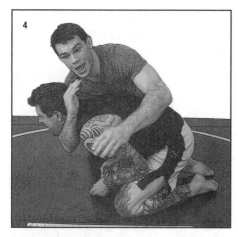

I seize the moment by wrapping my right arm around Neil's neck. I conclude this step of the technique by pulling my thumb out of his ass.

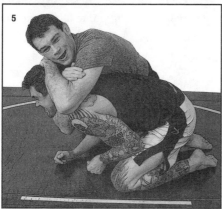

I grab my left biceps with my right hand, and then cup my left hand around the back of Neil's head.

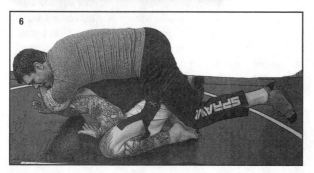

I climb onto Neil's back. To lock in the submission, I drive his head downward with my left hand and squeeze my arms tight. FYI, if your opponent sprawls lazily out on the mat and begins taking slow drags off a cigarette after you execute this technique, do not use it on him again.

KYOKOSHIKIN

I have to admit, a lot of the techniques in this section aren't supersecret, but this one absolutely is. As you know, I spent four years of my life living in a small Korean village, and it was there that a Zen master taught me this unbeatable move. It takes real dedication and months of your life to master, but it is well worth the investment, as it can be applied to the street, the cage, even when fighting underwater. Even though I've made a lot of cheap jokes throughout this book, I wanted you to walk away with something real and tangible. I have sacrificed the trust of many to share this with you, so please do not misuse this piece of fighting knowledge. If you look at the photos you'll notice that the most critical steps are two and three. It is very important that you get the hand positioning just right. You do not simply want to grab your opponent's elbow—you want to tweak it up and back. This will cause him severe pain, allowing you to latch onto his neck with your opposite hand and drive your left foot into his sternum. When executed with the proper form, the end result is what you see in photo 4.

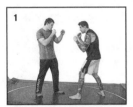

I'm squared off with Neil in my fighting stance.

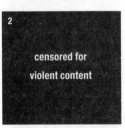

Neil throws a jab, and I immediately intercept it with my right hand, shoot my left hand underneath his right leg, and kick out his left knee. As he goes down, I grab his elbows with my hands and bend them over the back of his head, disrupting his balance and cutting off blood to his brain. Next, I wrap my right arm around the back of his neck, grab his left foot with my right hand, and force his left leg over his right shoulder. As you can see, this not only puts unbelievable pressure on his spine, but it also affects his vision.

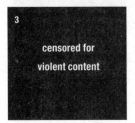

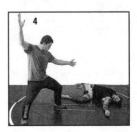

Without letting go of Neil's elbows, I drive my right knee down into his kidney, rendering him unconscious.

I back away.

EPILOGUE

For the handful of you who actually made it through this book, I feel I need to reward you in some way. I don't know where all of you live, so I can't mail you a chocolate-covered apple. And even if I did know where you all lived, sending a chocolate-covered apple might appear creepy, especially if you are a young child. So all I can really do is offer the other side of manliness, the side that was overlooked in this epic manifesto.

While being manly is certainly about fixing shit like heaters and your old lady's vibrator, it goes well beyond tinkering with extremely large mechanical devices. It's about being able to repair shit in your life and in the lives of others. It's about doing the right thing. You might ask yourself, What is the right thing? Unless you're a clinical-grade sociopath, you should know. Or at least you did when you were a kid. If something feels wrong and you have to look both ways before doing it, that shit is probably fucking wrong. For example, when I stole my cousin's G.I. Joe, it felt pretty wrong, and it was. If you've been so diluted by Japanese bukkake porn that you no longer know the difference between good and not good, following the basic tenets of any religion is an excellent place to start. I don't consider myself a religious person, and yet I pray. I pray that there is a God and that He is good. I want there to be a God so much, I don't give a damn which God it is. He could even be Asian. Seriously, if I die and go to heaven only to find a fat Asian at the Pearly Gates, as long as I get to rub His tummy, I won't be angry at anything.

I know what some of you might be thinking—religion can be a good thing, but it can also be seriously fucked up. There are two thoughts on this. The first thought comes from the philosopher Pascal. He was a serious pimp back in the day, and he believed that following the basic tenets of any religion would help us have a more functional and orderly society. This is true for the big-picture laws, such as do not kill or rape or piss on your neighbor's rose bushes, down to the smaller laws, such as don't eat pork. When we follow these laws, we are kind to one another and avoid trichinosis, which can be contracted by consuming swine. We live happier, more fulfilling lives. If you die and there is a God, you're stocked. If you kick the bucket and there is no God, at least you lived a healthy life.

On the opposite side, you have the atheist belief. If you're a follower of this philosophy, you believe that worshiping a god and following the rules of a specific church will detract from your life. Religion constricts your thinking, takes up a bunch of time you could have spent playing backgammon, and leads to wars that claim millions of lives. Personally, I choose Pascal's belief. I figure as long as I never kill in the name of a God, I'm good. However, I don't feel that you need to believe in a certain religion to be saved. The God I imagine doesn't demand you follow a certain script. He is happy as long as you are benevolent. As a result, I have built my religion much like how MMA was constructed—by picking things from different religions that work for me. I like the Ten Commandments (minus the one where you can't take the Lord's name in vain), and I like concepts from Buddhism. Of course, there is a downside because you may leave out some very important things, but it all goes back to common sense.

The only thing that I have had trouble with on this religious path of mine is if there really is a God, why would He let so many people suffer? The only answer I've come up with during those brief moments when my brain actually has had original thoughts was that it is the job of those of us who aren't suffering to help those who are. I know what you're probably thinking: What have you done to make the world a better place, Forrest? Other than helping out at the homeless shelter when I was fourteen, not that much. Well, this is your chance to be better than a UFC fighter. And I promise that I will try to reprioritize. You'll see. My most glorious moment, my Gandhi moment, will be when I take down Ann Coulter, Bill Maher, and Bill O'Reilly. Once I've done that, I will have done my part to make the world a better place.

—Forrest

P.S. If my epilogue seemed utterly retarded, that's because it was written by a retard. Seriously, my IQ is only seventeen points above retard level. I learned of this fact when I took an IQ test as a freshman in college. The lady who gave me the score didn't come out and say, "Boy, you're one stupid son of a bitch!" It was even worse because she broke it to me softly, much like a mother would when telling her five-year-old son that his dog has been chewed up by the plow.

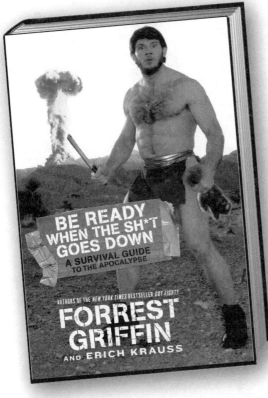